It all begins in the waiting room

July 27, 2015

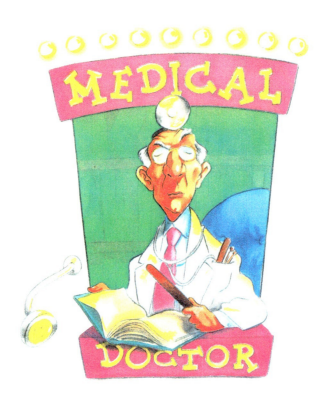

It all begins in the waiting room

How to drive your doctor crazy while escaping retaliation

Dr. David Rapoport

FUNNY DOC PUBLICATIONS

Copyright © David Rapoport, 2015
All rights reserved. No part of this book may be reproduced in any form or by any electronic or mechanical means, including information storage or retrieval systems, without permission of Funny Doc Publications. Reviewers, however, may quote brief passages in a review. Permissions to photocopy should be requested from Access Copyright.

Library and Archives Canada Cataloguing in Publication data

Rapoport, David, 1941-, author
    It all begins in the waiting room : how to drive your doctor crazy while escaping retaliation / Dr. David Rapoport.

Includes bibliographical references.
ISBN 978-0-9940895-0-2 (pbk.)

    1. Physician and patient—Humor. 2. Medicine—Humor. I. Title.

PN6231.M4R36 2015   C818'.602   C2015-902720-9

Editor: Rosemary Shipton
Proofreader: Judy Phillips
Author photograph: Sharon Rapoport
Design: Peter Ross / Counterpunch Inc.
Printing: IngramSpark

Funny Doc Publications
funnydoc@rogers.com

Illustration Credits
Care has been taken to trace the ownership of copyright material used in this book. The author and publisher welcome any information regarding errors or omissions.
Andy, 32
Gary Clement, front cover, 214
Peter Cook, 182
Tom Goldsmith, 17, 45, 134
Dave Prothero, 86, 142
Craig Terison, 168
Dave Whamond, 187, 202, 238

*To my late parents, Rose and
Louis Rapoport, and to my wife, Sharon*

Contents

Introduction   11

Staff
Staff – our first line of defence   16
Hurricane Mabel – my mixed-up medical secretary   18
Medical secretary required – ideal qualifications   21

Waiting-room adventures
Waiting, waiting, and more waiting – ten patients behind   30
A demented duo takes over the waiting room   35
Patients who fight   37
Thumps in the waiting room   39
Drop-in Bob   41

In the examining room
Goofy about gonads   43
The rear admiral   47
The window washer and the pelvic exam   49
Belly laughs   50
Punmeister   53
Emergencies – firefighters, police officers,
    and ambulance attendants   56
Lying in state in the doctor's office   58
The gamblers   60

Abominations and embarrassing situations
    How to make your physician remember you   66
    How to make your patients remember you   71

Tools of the trade
    Doctors causing high blood pressure   75
    The stethoscope – the colder the better   78
    The many uses of the humble tongue depressor   80
    The nerd pocket   82

Peculiar patients
    Doorknobs, handshakes, and other hazards   85
    Examining-room ballet   90
    Fainters, grabbers, and smoochers   92
    The carrot people   95
    Whistlers and hummers   97

Physicians' bad habits
    Performing ritual Sudoku in medical practice   101
    The five-pound Hershey bar   105
    Snoozing sickness   108
    Snoozing physicians   111
    Doctors who yell   115
    Hiccups   118

Mind games
    Beware of honest physicians – they may be dangerous   122
    Bizarre coincidences in medical practice   126
    Deconstructing Michelangelo's *David*   128

Drug reps, drug companies, and prescription pads

    Drug reps bearing flattery, adulation, and praise   133

    Drug companies bearing gifts   137

    Drug dreams   140

    A daring method of drug selection for the harried family physician   145

    Goldilocks revisited   149

    Reconstructing Mary   152

    My polydoctor patient   156

    A cautionary tale about vultures, fish, snakes, and devils on drugs   158

Meeting patients outside the office

    House calls – how to handle dogs, doors, and defunct doorbells   162

    Lessons in patient avoidance   164

    The beach, the mall, and the wedding hall   166

    Is there a doctor on the plane?   170

Doctors get sick too

    Coronary heart disease   173

    Sleep apnea   177

Baseball as metaphor for the practice of medicine

    Doctors and baseball pitchers must get the opponent out   183

    A new seasonal affective disorder   186

Body image and plastic surgery

    The widow's facelift   191

    Why plastic surgery patients switch doctors   193

    My nude dye job   197

    Bald and balder – or a tale of two drug reps   199

    Big-belly syndrome   203

Sex
  Fleeing from temptation   207
  Viagra – making sex fun at any age   209

Parents and elderly patients
  My parents – our waiting-room spies   213
  Death takes a holiday   220
  Logistical problems in treating the elderly   223
  Driving while demented   226
  Vehicular attack – good golly, it's Dolly!   229
  Accident-prone people   231

Endings – doctors and patients
  Firing a doctor, firing a patient, and transferring records   235
  Olfactory adventures   239

New beginnings
  Rating MDs – how to fight back   243
  Electronic medical records   246
  Capitation and its temptations   249

  About the author   252
  Acknowledgements   253
  Credits   254

Introduction

In our daily work as family physicians we may face contagion, accusations, and naked displays of aggression and misshapen bodies. We have booby-trapped brown bags full of drugs and other strange things dumped on our desks. Hypochondriacs, malcontents, malingerers, and neurotic and seductive patients appear in much higher proportions in our offices than in other professions, and they challenge us daily.

Many stories are found in the section "Peculiar patients." Every visit may be a skirmish if you are one of those patients who inadvertently cause doctors discomfort or fear, as in the examples in the section "Abominations and embarrassing situations." Once the door to the examining room is closed and we are alone with the patient, the fun begins.

We must match wits with patients who want us to arrange three different specialists each time they come in. Others twist our arms unless we prescribe unnecessary drugs or order CT scans or MRIs for minor problems. One of these individuals is described in the chapter "My polydoctor patient." We also contend with highly skilled double-doctoring drug addicts in search of narcotics. Some of my patients have been very creative in this regard, but we can always dump them, as I describe in the section "Endings."

Fortunately, physicians have some secret defences and bad habits, as you'll see in the section "Mind games" or in my surprising use of Sudoku as a relief. In our efforts to survive with our dignity and health intact, we physicians employ some ancient and modern techniques, mainly but not always painless, harmless, and undetected.

There are three key individuals in the cast of characters in this drama: the medical secretary, the physician, and the patient.

Another featured actor is the ominously growling waiting room, where five to fifteen other patients wait nervously and sometimes angrily. Consultants can also be bad actors at times, including the "Rear admiral" and the "Snoozing physician."

The first contact between the patient and the doctor is the phone call to book an appointment. If "Hurricane Mabel" is on duty, prepare for chaos because she has never solved the mysteries of the two-line phone. You may be cut off before you speak. On arrival, note that the waiting room is usually crowded. Look around at your fellow patients who come and go. Read some of the strategy our usually efficient receptionists employ in dealing with the more assertive and theatrical examples in "Staff – our first line of defence." Be on the alert while in the waiting room because strange things might be happening which are hazardous to the innocent person reading quietly in the corner. The most bizarre experiences are detailed in the section "Waiting-room adventures."

In the section "Tools of the trade," I explain how I use some of our common objects in surprising ways, including tongue depressors and stethoscopes. Simple blood-pressure measurements can involve a war of nerves that the doctor often loses. My prescription pad is placed on the desk between the patient and me like the loaded weapon it truly is. The visit often ends with a race to control the all-important doorknob, as described in the section "Peculiar patients." Money-laundering occasionally takes place when I arrive home with my "nerd pocket" full to bursting, but that is more innocent than it sounds.

Patients may wonder if the healer is paying any attention to their woeful tales. A vacant look means that your doctor is thinking about lunch as you relate a story he or she has likely heard hundreds of times before. If he falls completely asleep during the visit, there are opportunities for mayhem, as I discuss in two "snoozing" stories. If you feel annoyed and would like to express your frustration in a confrontational way, you can savage your doctor's reputation anonymously by scoring him low in various categories on the RateMDs website. He has ways to retaliate once he figures out which patient sent in the rating.

The section "Drugs" reviews all the aspects of our most potent weapon, the prescribing of drugs. How do we choose from a bewildering assortment of copycat drugs, similar in so many respects? Simple: at times I prescribe only those drugs that begin with the letters *A* and *Z*. Pharmaceutical companies and their drug reps are quite influential in this matter, and I discuss them at length.

Do we doctors know what we are doing with drugs? Sadly, we often do not, and that is the subject of "Deconstructing Michelangelo's *David*," in which this famous and handsome towering individual is turned into a toxic-waste dump by an envious and evil physician. "Reconstructing Mary" sets things right. For examples of harmful doctors on a smaller scale, read the stories grouped together in the section "Mind games."

The section "Sex" deals with both the seductive patient and the lustful physician because, sadly, some exist of both genders. You'll also find here the important issue of Viagra and low testosterone levels, or "Low T," in men. The section "Body image and plastic surgery" reviews common requests from patients for procedures such as facelifts, penile implants, and bariatric surgery.

I discuss termination of the unique connection family physicians have with patients in the section "Endings." If you want to fire your doctor after you read this book, you should learn that the doctor may fire you first. Retirement of the physician leads to many issues, especially to the question of who owns the medical records you have watched your doctor studiously scribble down at every visit. Finding a new physician has become somewhat easier now that family practice is enjoying a resurgence.

Finally, in the section "New beginnings" I describe two very controversial innovations in my practice. In "Electronic medical records" I describe EMRs as a mixed blessing. Initially they make eye contact quite difficult as most older MDs struggle with their new computer monitors and printers, but they soon enough become comfortable with the system. In "Capitation and its temptations" you'll learn how doctors can be paid for *not* seeing patients. The end of the fee-for-service system is altering medical practice in many ways. I explain here how my robotic medical assistant Oscar has the ability to replace my human staff – and why I fear he is close to replacing me.

STAFF

Staff – our first line of defence

I have the greatest admiration and sympathy for the countless thousands of nurses, hospital workers, and medical secretaries and receptionists who work directly with patients. I have employed many wonderful women in my office over the years and remain on a first-name basis with secretaries who have worked for my colleagues as well.

They do have their limits, however. I recently learned that Joyce, a small and delightful sixty-year-old, was so ticked off after an argument that she grabbed the offending man by the collar and marched him right out of her office. One of my own secretaries once took accusations and verbal abuse over the phone for five minutes before she flushed crimson, slowly stood up, and began to snort. Then she exploded and unleashed a vocabulary of swear words. As I listened in awe she told the man she had never heard such a load of garbage from any human being in the seven years she had worked in my office – and promptly slammed down the phone. I knew the patient could have this effect on people, so I settled her down and congratulated her. In the aftermath, I fired the patient but kept her.

Physicians could not possibly do such work themselves without committing murder or mayhem, as I discovered numerous times when a receptionist was ill. Mostly it's a female profession: women are better at multitasking and dealing with children, and many adult patients revert to childhood – tantrums included. Help-wanted ads cannot specify gender, but after many years of talking to my colleagues' secretaries, only twice has a man answered the phone. One was the spouse of the doctor, and I suspect that the other was a woman with a deep voice. Men may be completely unsuitable for this kind of work.

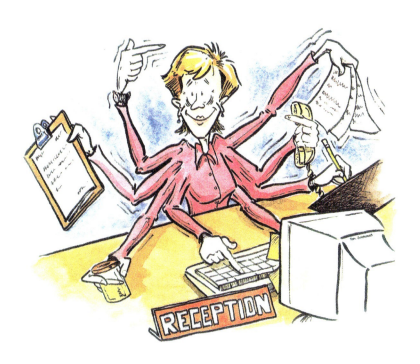

Hurricane Mabel – my mixed-up medical secretary

Something quite unusual and disturbing was going on in our waiting room. Unlike the quiet hum I normally hear as patients come and go, I heard loud voices and uproarious laughter. I peeked out to see that Mabel, my new secretary/receptionist of mature years, had caused several serious breaches of waiting-room etiquette.

Unwritten rules of the medical office make it clear that patients must not speak to each other in this anxiety-provoking situation. Yet here they were, not only talking but enjoying back-slapping merriment at Mabel's expense. Furthermore, patients generally do not even look at each other as they wait, except for a brief glance while finding a safe seat. They maintain their privacy by reading, with heads down. This time, however, they were revelling in the camaraderie of this novel experience.

The most important rule in a medical office states that prudent staff must not enter a busy waiting room, for fear of confrontation with patients. But brave little Mabel, clipboard and pen in hand, was doing the rounds from person to person, forgetting which ones she had already "greeted." It was obvious that Mabel could not keep them in the correct order, and some were becoming quite angry.

Fortunately for her, when the phone rang, she escaped from this den. Unfortunately for me, Mabel knew nothing about telephone etiquette either. It requires prompt attention to each caller, and the polite and efficient use of the "hold" button where necessary. To my chagrin, I saw that Mabel had not mastered the concept of putting one line on hold while she dealt with the other when it rang. She cut several people off, and generally confused patients and pharmacists. As a result, pharmacists could not get medication renewed, the sick could not make appointments, and referrals to other physicians or for tests had to wait. Routines such as filing lab results and pulling charts were also problematic for her as she fluttered about nervously, clacking her false teeth and mumbling to herself.

Mabel was very eager to look good on that first day on the job, especially when my associate Dr. Martin and I were around, so she repeatedly dashed out to the expectant group in the waiting room. Perhaps she was trying to escape our frowns as we shook our heads in disbelief. In any case, we saw and heard the crowd growing and growling ominously, as "office gridlock" developed. More patients were arriving, but no one was leaving, because Dr. Martin and I had stopped working while trying to get Mabel organized. New arrivals could barely enter the office. Some sat in the corridor until they got used to the hilarity, then joined in the fun.

Mabel's desire to please led to a most embarrassing incident: she indecently exposed herself to us at a typical moment of high anxiety. While we were talking to her, she dropped something on the floor. As we all bent over to pick it up, nearly knocking heads, she stepped on the back hem of her dress. Immediately she lost her balance, fell flat on her back, with legs akimbo in the air, and offered us a full view of her antiquated knickers. I helped her up and pretended not to have seen anything. Without a pause, Mabel was up and off again in her destructive routine.

At day's end, we surveyed the smoking battlefield. Our confused patients had all struggled out, files were piled everywhere, urine samples had spilled, and lab reports had been thrown out unread. Mabel had garbled the messages of the few callers who had succeeded in getting through to us. Large gaps were present in our schedules for the next day because frustrated callers had not been able to make appointments.

It was obvious I had made a grave error in offering Mabel the job. My motive was noble – I was trying to hire someone who was quite a bit older than the rest of us in my medical office. To compound Mabel's distress and our own, I gave her extra time to learn the job, but she never did master the two-line phone or many other simple tasks. Finally, a cousin, who was also my patient, convinced me to let her go, after describing some outrageous scenes in my waiting room. I have never found it easy to fire someone, but Mabel should have gone weeks before. I deliberated for a few days, and then she made things easier by quitting.

What is Mabel doing now, fully ten years later? Her next job was volunteering in the medical records department of my local hospital, where she lasted several years. We had parted as friends, and she always greeted me pleasantly whenever I had to do a dictation. Our hospital still achieved its accreditation in spite of misplaced charts and documents.

More recently, Mabel has been doing volunteer work in our reception and outpatient departments. She is the first staff person people see when they enter our hospital. Her job is to direct traffic, and her desk is usually surrounded by people shaking their heads. When I see confused individuals wandering around our corridors, I know she is on duty. Mabel is a kind and good soul, but she is still the picture of incompetence, flitting around in her pink volunteer outfit, mumbling and clacking her teeth. Her supervisor must be too kind to let her go. No doubt she will soon be volunteering in some other department.

Medical secretary required – ideal qualifications

Long after Mabel left, I still had occasional disasters with receptionists: one of them wore shorts to the office and grew to like the smell of photocopier fluid; another tied up our office phones with personal calls. One bold woman yelled at me and refused to include me in tea time after my innocent quip about a previous cup of tea. A temporary employee who filled in for a single day announced, "This is a job for three people." Sadly, one receptionist became psychotic, but I like to think she had such tendencies before she was hired.

My new associate, Dr. Susan, and I decided to draw up a list of qualifications we considered necessary for a medical secretary at the time. I'll deal with the physical and educational requirements separately, starting with the first. Hazards are also included.

SIZE AND STRENGTH: Pam, our last secretary, exceeded our five-feet-minimum height requirements, enabling her to reach the fifth level of our lateral filing cabinets. She was also slender, which prevented some accidents in our narrow corridors. This point is important: Dr. Susan is also thin but moves at lightning speed, while my elderly patients and I are often dawdling in the hallway, making collisions inevitable. The secretary is expected to bounce right back up and, though winded, assist everybody to their feet, before collecting patients' false teeth and canes.

WEIGHT LIFTING: Pam, unfortunately, lacked upper-body strength on her small frame. She needed our help hauling male patients over to an examining table after they collapsed to the floor after a venipuncture or allergy shot. Dr. Susan and I come running if we hear the characteristic thud, but the secretary is on her own if she grabs the patient before he hits the ground.

MARTIAL ARTS TRAINING: Besides strength, a medical secretary should have boxing and wrestling skills: the first to referee and separate waiting-room combatants during scuffles over "Who's next?" and the last to help manhandle powerful children who do not want to be examined. We doctors restrain the upper body and head, but Pam had trouble controlling the squirming pelvis and kicking feet. Judo and karate skills are useful in dealing with male flirts who sense an opportunity to practise their suggestive patter or even fondle someone who they feel cannot escape or slap them in the face. This group includes men who are half nude or even in their Jockey shorts while having an ECG. An elbow to the nose or a judo-chop to the neck helps here, with a knee to the groin held in reserve.

SECURITY TRAINING: The modern secretary is the front line of defence against unbalanced patients or those with a grudge about some failed treatment. Many strange characters wander in and out of every medical office, and she must know how to stare down rowdy types and deflect their anger. At the very least, she must distract them and hold them back while the rest of us escape through the back door. Sadly, two Canadian physicians have been shot in recent years, so she might consider wearing a bulletproof vest.

ASSERTIVENESS TRAINING AND CHILDREN'S DAY-CARE EXPERIENCE: Firmness and fortitude are needed to handle theatrical patients who plead for non-existing appointments, scolds who complain about long waits or some other discomfort, and chatterboxes who usurp the secretary's attention, keeping her away from her work despite entreaties to "please take a seat." For the same reasons, experience with children helps to organize the ever-changing kindergarten of ten or fifteen adult patients in the office at any given time. It is commonly known that people revert to childhood when they are sick, especially the men, so she must distract them with magazines and insist on "quiet times" if the noise level becomes excessive.

CONTAMINATED WASTE MANAGEMENT: The secretary must live with constant bombardments of bacteria and viruses. For some reason, the most infectious patients often ask to use her phone. Nervous Pam began toward the end of her tenure with us to wear a mask, lab coat, and gloves while on duty. We physicians are responsible for sorting our contaminated waste, but Pam was terrified she might get a needle prick from a syringe used on someone with AIDS or hepatitis A, B, or C.

THE GAGGING FACTOR: "I'm not cleaning it up!" said Pam, when we heard a patient retching in our washroom. This retreat summed up her attitude to the disgusting things that occur in every medical office. Pam also tried not to peek while assisting us during pelvic exams. She passed equipment while peering out between the fingers covering her eyes, so she constantly dropped speculums, which then had to be sterilized again. The prudent male physician can no longer be left alone for these personal examinations, so Pam's behaviour became a big problem. The secretary's presence prevents a patient's future complaints of sexual abuse.

And now for the educational and experience qualifications.

MEDICAL OFFICE EXPERIENCE: Previous experience is invaluable when the medical secretary has to decide while talking to a patient over the phone who should come to the office, who needs a house call, and who should hasten to the nearest hospital emergency department. Dr. Susan and I try not to make phone calls while seeing other patients, so we expect the secretary to handle most requests for health advice about minor problems. We need someone with considerable experience in practising medicine without a licence – the kind of knowledge gained from many previous years in a family practice office.

PHONE EXPERIENCE: The phones are always busy with appointment seekers, many of whom will be unhappy with the time offered. Other patients call asking for results, which means their charts have to be pulled. Still others demand to speak to the doctor, and these rude folk often refuse to divulge the reason for their concern. We doctors get annoyed by these demands, and we call back later, when we have time, or perhaps we "forget" to place the call to aggressive patients. Unfortunately, it's easy for doctors to transfer this irritation onto the secretary, partly because at noon or long after their day should have ended they are exhausted, thirsty, hungry, hypoglycaemic, and overstimulated mentally after solving patient problems, making referrals, and writing prescriptions, all with a smile.

Calls from outside physicians, visiting nurses, or social workers must be directed at once to the doctor, while other doctors' secretaries need to be contacted to arrange appointments, obtain results, or play telephone tag, as neither employer is usually available when needed. There are times when the receptionist seems to have a phone stuck permanently on the side of her face. After a couple of hours, when the receptionist is ready to verbally decapitate anyone else who dares to phone, the next caller is invariably her employer's spouse.

PHARMACY EDUCATION: The secretary will spend half her time dealing with the renewal of drugs, up to fifteen for each patient, requested by any of the fifty local pharmacists and their staffs. Dr. Susan and I prescribe over a hundred different medications, most of which are impossible for an untrained person to pronounce or spell, and each must be written in the file. There is usually some urgency in repeating prescriptions because patients may have completely run out of something. Most often it is because they are nagging the pharmacist, who turns to our receptionist for relief. Dr. Susan and I, resenting phone interruptions during appointments, must be grabbed literally in the brief window of opportunity as we move between examining rooms.

HOSTESS: Every hour, our receptionist has to greet eight or ten patients, most of whom are anxious about the visit and irritable. Some come early and some late, and some have no appointment at all but fib and say they do. Some need follow-up visits or tests and referrals to be arranged. Some patients are overly friendly and perch in the secretary's window, looking for conversation and keeping her from her work. Some are scolds who are abusive about appointments and delays. The most aggressive ask other patients about the time of their appointments and pace around, settling down in front of the office door. Yet the customer is always right.

COMEDIENNE EXPERIENCE: This training will help the medical secretary engage in "gallows humour" with us about patients and enable her to cheer us up when the going gets tough and we can't remember why we wanted to get into this stressful career in the first place. We have agreed to do our guffawing behind closed doors so the patients don't hear us. As all physicians learn, patients waiting in the office misinterpret laughter and think we are laughing at them. The secretary must also be discreet enough to avoid humour when we docs are in very black moods and unapproachable. That happens to all physicians, when things go badly with a patient's health or after a disagreement with a patient.

PSYCHIC ABILITY: This sixth sense is invaluable in finding lost charts, saving those frustrating hours spent searching for them. If the secretary can probe my cerebrum, she might find that I took the file home to do a report. Mind reading also helps when I am hovering nearby as she handles calls on both lines and deals with patients coming and going. She won't waste time wondering, "What could he possibly want now, when he sees how busy I am?"

ANGER MANAGEMENT: Control plays a key role here, as the busy office day progresses. In truth, anyone with little self-control might go berserk and start throwing and breaking things. Dr. Susan and I add to the anger-load by beeping our medical secretary via our intercom system at random intervals. This sound is too annoying to ignore. Because she has two employers but only two hands, her urge to turn these hands into fists at times is quite understandable. Some patients can be extremely rude to medical office staff, but these same discourteous folk become angelic when finally in the presence of the doctor: "Don't worry about keeping me waiting," they say. "I'm retired – I've got all day."

COMPUTER SKILLS: The secretary must know how to use our computer for word processing and billing – a skill that is taught over several semesters of college or business school. Yet we somehow expect staff to learn how to do these complicated tasks on the job, in a two-hour lesson, while attending to other office problems. There is a Catch-22 here: most secretaries old enough to be experienced in medical offices are terrified of computers, treating them like bombs about to go off if the keyboard is touched. It is inhumane to expect people over the age of forty to suffer such computer-angst, but it must be done. Recently we began using electronic medical records in our office, and, fortunately, both secretaries handled this transition well with minimum training.

PSYCHOTHERAPY AND COUNSELLING QUALIFICATIONS: Some authorities believe that over half the patients who visit family physicians have anxiety or stress as the basis of their problems. They must receive a sympathetic greeting and be handled with care, or they take offence. To make things worse, many such patients express their hidden anger by impatient badgering of the secretary. They are tough to love. Everyone who applies for the position of medical secretary should prepare for the worst-case scenario, which in family practice happens often. I clearly remember finding one former receptionist spinning in circles, saying, "I don't know what to do first." I had to sit her down while she got herself sorted out. Another young woman at busy times would stand crouched like a football fullback behind her desk, hands apart, ready for anything and contemplating her next play. She seemed to feel that she had to be ready to charge past a patient and go deep for a forward pass when I called her from my office.

While all this activity is taking place, I am usually doing my own job, oblivious far behind the front lines. When I emerge at noon or 5 p.m. and see my shell-shocked helper, my innocent comment may be, "Quiet today, eh? Not too many problems. Have the phones been busy?" Fortunately, exhausted by that time, my secretary cannot throw anything at me.

To summarize the qualifications we need for our superhuman medical secretary: we want an athletic woman with a firm manner and a strong stomach. She must be able to work in a dangerous environment. She must be an intelligent and sensitive woman, with medical, nursing, pharmacy, and therapist skills. She must be computer-literate and able to work in a busy and noisy environment with demanding patients and employers. Previous experience is essential. Salary is negotiable, but usually abominable.

WAITING-ROOM ADVENTURES

Waiting, waiting, and more waiting – ten patients behind

Chaos reigned on the third floor of our medical building one morning. Down at our end of the corridor were two noisy children and several men and women, grouped anxiously outside our office door. Any newly arrived patient getting off the elevator who dared to pass through this gauntlet entered a waiting room with ten occupied seats and a lineup of folks in front of our receptionist's desk. Phones were ringing, a child was screaming, some people were grumbling loudly, and I was wishing I was somewhere else – anywhere else.

Our secretary Maria, bless her, had this unusual situation well in hand, saying, "Please take a seat if you can find one, we will get to you in order." Because every seat was taken, new arrivals could choose between leaning against a wall or joining the corridor crowd. Some joked in earnest, asking, "Should I take a number?" before commiserating with fellow sufferers. No one was happy, least of all my associate Dr. Susan and I, occasionally spotted clutching patient files and dashing nervously between examining rooms.

Amazingly, by 1 p.m. everyone had been seen and sent home or off to labs, consultants, hospital, or drugstores. But some had waited an hour for their turn in this organized confusion – something that happens occasionally in every medical office. In spite of all the turmoil, that morning finished not much later than any other, as is usually the case.

Fortunately, waiting rooms are usually quiet and less crowded, but they remain places of anxiety. Patients pretend to appear uninterested in the clock or in the order of patients being seen, but they are very aware if the doctor is running behind. Most expect and will tolerate a short wait. After a long wait, however, our more aggressive patients demonstrate restaurant lineup behaviour, standing up to ask our secretary how long they should expect to wait and how many people are ahead of them. Some of them stand at the entrance to the consulting rooms, blocking the passage and ready to hop in as soon as their turn comes. Some will question others about the appointment time they were given. Maddening to the already agitated is the fact that when both doctors are working, they can't assess whether someone is called out of turn.

What these bad actors cannot know is that Dr. Susan and I are fully aware of their behaviour and that our own frustration levels rise with the number of people waiting. And we certainly don't appreciate patients who scold our receptionist and pace around in the waiting room, disturbing others who are sitting quietly and reading.

When a particularly large and unruly mob has formed, we docs prudently abandon the time-honoured custom of peeking into the waiting room to call the next patient in, for fear of being accosted. Our secretaries get this pleasure, for which they should receive danger pay. Many hopeful bottoms rise a bit from their chairs in expectation whenever Maria looks out, but only one is called. The others go plop in resignation.

Once I have said hello to my patient in the examination room and made my apologies, sensible folks often comment, "No problem, doc, you are very busy today." These words are code for "You sure kept me waiting a long time today. My time is valuable too, you know."

It makes no sense to antagonize one's physician on the subject of delays, but some fools do, saying angrily, "You kept me an hour out there. I can't take that when I go to a doctor." Most likely they arrived thirty minutes before the appointment time, so the long wait is half their own fault. In voicing their chagrin they disturb the very person who is about to make critical decisions regarding their health and may even perform a procedure or give an injection, thereby inviting a perfect opportunity to exact revenge.

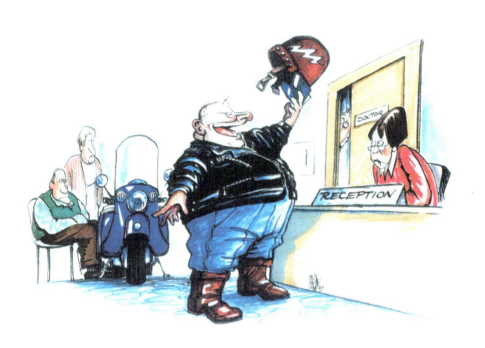

Whatever, doctors do have long memories, and rude remarks to staff or to us do not sit well. After many years in practice, I generally just listen and nod when confronted by a complainer, but I have my favourite rejoinders at the ready, if I am sufficiently bothered. With a tight smile I tell my difficult patient, "I am delayed because I have been attending to patients who need more time, as you may some day. Emergencies happen. I think you can tell that I have not been on a long coffee break." An effective alternative is to say, "I can send you to a different doctor down the street who will not keep you waiting – he graduated three weeks ago."

A really harassed physician might snap back, "If you don't like it, go find another doctor and don't bother me again!" Most of us never treat patients with such rudeness, but we all have several characters we would dearly love to lose.

Somehow, even on bad days, things usually get sorted out without any arguments, and every patient is seen. As a bonus to the tired physician, after a very long wait, most patients shorten their lists of complaints. They want to escape and see the light of day, and generally they are delighted to have a speedy visit. Some even leave while I'm still talking!

And what about the healer? There must be a short mid-morning and mid-afternoon break to refuel and answer urgent phone calls. I find that eating an apple at these times does the trick nicely – somehow, you can't rush an apple. Amazingly, in their efforts to stay on time, few docs I know take such a break. Nor did I, until my own physician told me to do so. Physicians are geared up by training to work past the point of exhaustion.

Why do family physicians get behind? Most of us budget fifteen minutes per patient, or four per hour, which makes for a full and comfortable schedule of prearranged appointments. Invariably, other patients will phone with legitimate acute problems and need an appointment, becoming the fifth person for each hour. That's my personal maximum – or I become a patient.

While some visits are brief, others take longer, when patients have more complicated problems such as chest pain, abdominal pain, or dizzy spells. The careful physician must now rule out coronary heart disease, a surgical problem, or a brain tumour. Each such visit can take up to thirty minutes. One bedlam day we had to resuscitate a patient who was having a coronary and deal with ambulance attendants, police, and the fire department, but new arrivals didn't know what had happened.

Everyone seems to be under stress these days, creating anxiety, insomnia, and depression. If patients want to talk about these problems, we must listen and advise them, and these consultations take still more time. Any opportunity to help a reticent patient must not be lost.

Understandably, most physicians are sensitive to the patients in the waiting room, and we share their irritation. We are mainly type-A personalities ourselves, and we would dearly love to run on schedule. But this luxury is clearly impossible in our profession. My best advice to patients in the lineup is to bring a book and a healthy attitude when you come for an appointment – and an apple for the doctor too.

A demented duo takes over the waiting room

We Canadians are generally a reserved bunch, and we do not usually speak to strangers, whether in a subway, restaurant, or elevator. Anyone who starts a conversation is looked at with suspicion. This custom certainly applies in a doctor's waiting room, where the guy in the next seat might have a contagious disorder or be a little peculiar.

One day, however, the sound of a horn honking and one man laughing while another was shouting told me that the impossible had happened. Sam and Lou, my partly demented and mildly psychotic patients, had arrived in my waiting room at the same hour and were meeting each other for the first time. My secretary and I looked into the room and saw that our other patients were equally stunned. Sloppy Sam and his horn had an appointment, but dapper Lou did not: we generally take care not to book two disruptive patients in the same hour. Worse, Lou had escaped from the supervision of his wife, the only person able to control him.

Sam had arrived first, dressed in layers of clothing like a homeless person and honking a child's toy horn. He further annoyed others with offers of candy and comments, and addressed a comely young woman with the words, "Well, well, what have we here? You are a real beauty. Hubba, hubba, come sit beside me." Sam's psychiatrist described him best, in psycho-jargon, as being "extremely jocular and quite loud ... very intrusive and sexually inappropriate."

At that moment the elegant Lou arrived, as usual holding a briefcase full of his writings. Sam announced Lou's arrival with his horn, and said, "Hello, professor: Welcome, have a seat!" They became fast friends, because Lou knew a good audience when he saw one, and he handed Sam and everyone else in the waiting room copies of his work. Despite Lou's sophisticated manner, my other patients knew he was strange as soon as he started shaking hands and asking for their names. He then began a lecture on world issues. Once finished, Lou was honked loudly by his new friend and applauded very tentatively by one or two others.

Lou shared Sam's unfortunate habit of commenting on and embarrassing strangers. If someone looked worried, he said so and tried to cheer him up. If an elderly woman had wrinkles, he said so and suggested wrinkle cream or a facelift. Lou had actually been arrested once, when a woman in a bank lineup took offence after he called her fat and helpfully suggested a diet. The judge in this case was lenient when he read my explanatory letter about Lou's "normal pressure hydrocephalus," a condition causing such behaviour. Sam had reached the same point by suffering from "multi-infarct dementia" caused by mini-strokes.

On the fateful day they met, my nurse and I separated these kindred spirits as soon as possible and gave both prompt attention, to restore peace to my office. Messy Sam went on to purchase a motor scooter, and he startled and embarrassed me on several occasions in our local shopping plaza by quietly scooting up behind me and tooting his loud cycle horn. Many other times he made a grand fuss when we met in the neighbourhood bank or bakery, announcing to all that I was his family physician. When Sam was admitted to a chronic-care facility, I received a desperate call from the physician in charge. Sam's antics had persisted, as I knew from her despairing tone and the background sounds of his horn and colourful language.

I last saw Sam in my acute-care hospital, where he died from his last stroke, but I was startled one last time a few days later when I was called to my phone and he was on the line. It was his son, thanking me for my efforts. He had Sam's exact tone, diction, and jocularity, and fortunately for me he lived in California, so no more reincarnations are expected. By then, the debonair Lou had also deteriorated and resided in a nursing home, where, to his delight, he had a captive audience.

Patients who fight

Anything can happen in a family physician's waiting room, where several thousand patients pass through every year. Fortunately, a serious patient-patient fight broke out only once in my office, and, for embarrassing reasons, I was helpless to stop it. Ironically, surgery was required later to reconstruct one participant's nose.

Helen and Sally were at the forty-five-minute stage in my waiting room when they got nasty with each other. Seventy-year-old Helen was visually impaired – and over the years I've found that vision- and hearing-challenged persons get more confused in the waiting-room chaos and need to be reassured that all is well. Helen was a suspicious and difficult woman. She was one of my very few patients, and the only female one, who used profanities during office visits. I didn't like that at all, but at the time I tolerated it. Much younger Sally, aged forty, was normally a pleasant person but had been anxious in recent months because of her mother's recent death after a long illness. Also on that day, she had to pick up her children from school by a certain fast-approaching time.

When my secretary asked, "Who's next?" I was occupied in my washroom, which is adjacent to the waiting room. I was only about three feet and one wall away from the spot where the altercation began as both ladies answered the call. I was able to hear the argument escalating but could not intervene, being midstream as it were. In my younger days, before the aging process caused some urinary hesitancy, perhaps this story would have a different ending.

Helen filled the air with obscenities, including "You *&%$#@, get out of my way, I'm next" and "Shut up or I'll knock your *&%$#@ teeth down your *&%$#@ throat." Sally retaliated and meanly pointed out that "old ladies have all the time in the world." I listened helplessly as tearful Sally then drew out her truly powerful weapon: she deserved special consideration, she said, because she had just lost her mother. Helen, without a pause, shot back: "Who cares? I lost my mother too" – and cited a date from forty years before!

By then I was quite alarmed and nearly had a dreadful accident while zipping up. I feared I might find my two patients rolling on the floor and locked in a hair-pulling embrace. Did I have local anaesthetic and suture material? Would the X-ray department in my building still be open to check for fractures? Would my secretary or my other patients get beaten up if they intervened? Was Helen using her stout cane to administer whacks? Does office insurance cover beatings? Should I call 911 to bring the police and paramedics? Things sounded very frightening from where I was standing.

Mercifully, no punches or shoves had taken place, and both appeared rather sheepish when I later examined them. I made the decision to take Sally first. Things could have been worse – Helen has since gone on to use her cane to hit a neighbour. She now feels that even her children are persecuting her. She still swears in my presence, even though I told her it made me uncomfortable. Her diagnosis: paranoid schizophrenia.

As for Sally's nose ... it was a purely cosmetic rhinoplasty. It caused me some embarrassment because I didn't recognize her at her next visit. She left my practice soon after, deciding to change her physician as well as her nose. More likely, she associated me with her mother's long and difficult illness and death, and she wanted a fresh start.

Thumps in the waiting room

We physicians are a hardy lot. We can take major stress without showing it to colleagues, staff, or patients, but my own ability to stay calm failed miserably with thirty-year-old Donald. It has taken several years for me to be able to tell this tale, and the passage of time has enabled me to see some humour in it.

Imagine a busy waiting room with patients coming and going, keeping my secretary occupied. Then picture me, deep in concentration with a patient, not twenty feet from the scene of the coming catastrophe. Relaxed, not even aware that Donald was out there (he had walked in without an appointment), I heard a sickening thump. That's all – no commotion, no distress calls from my secretary, just that thump. Thinking that someone must have dropped something in a nearby office or corridor, I carried on for ten more minutes. To my surprise, I found Donald in a post-seizure state sitting in my waiting room. His epileptic seizure had been strong enough to push his knee nearly through a wall. Shocked by this turn of events, I assessed Donald and advised him to alter his medication. His knee and other anatomical parts were fine, but my office wall looked as though a cannonball had hit it, with its broken drywall and wallpaper exposing the pipes and wires inside the cavity.

Meanwhile, Donald kept seeing me regularly. For the good of his health and my own sanity, I instituted the "Donald treatment." It goes as follows: When he makes an appointment, the time is circled in red. He is reminded the day before and is called if he doesn't show up, to avoid a surprise visit on another day. When Donald arrives, I am to be informed immediately. I excuse myself from the patient currently being examined and go to the other examining room to see him. When we are done, my secretary escorts him to the elevator to make sure he is all right. Whew! That is some job, but we do it, and everyone except the half-dressed patient I must run away from is happy.

After five uneventful years, we let the Donald treatment lapse. Sure enough, another thump soon followed. I was shocked again, but at least I knew what had happened and how to help him. Donald was fine soon after this second seizure, but I observed him for a while before he left, accompanied by family and carrying a stronger prescription. Only at the end of the day, as I left my office, did I notice that my wall had been defaced again – and in the same spot. Donald had pulled off the armrest of his chair and dug it into the wall during his seizure, forming a triangular gouge. Fortunately, this time the hole was big enough to be noticed, but not bad enough for the renovation routine. That meant looking at it until painting and wallpapering were next due.

The Donald treatment can be used for other waiting patients, such as the very ill or those with communicable diseases, and it can be valuable for eccentrics who disturb others. Do I still see Donald? Of course, but with the full treatment rigorously applied. He is healthy, but all his visits to my office are big events. Even if he were royalty, I could not do more for him. Seeing him immediately at least prevents his office seizures – and eliminates those dreaded thumps.

Drop-in Bob

After my patients' marriage broke up with much acrimony, Sue left my practice. I continued to see Bob, a rather rough sixty-year-old. As a city employee, he had a laid-back approach to the work ethic. He was also one of the most dreaded patients a physician can have: the guy who shows up without an appointment.

To my surprise, Sue phoned me five years later. She told me she wanted to return to my practice, with one condition: I had to assure her that she would not bump into Bob in my waiting room. That was a problem. I explained that her ex-spouse arrived any time he felt like it, though only in the afternoon, after making a token appearance at his job. Sue arranged a morning visit.

Sue had changed in that her vision was poor – a good thing as it turned out. She arrived on the appointed morning, and the waiting room filled up slowly as she sat in a corner. To the distress of my secretary and me, in walked Bob. He had decided to take the whole day off this time. In his usual way, he wanted to be seen immediately, but he realized that many fellow sufferers had preceded him. He looked slowly around, stopping just short of Sue, who thankfully could not see him well. He exited, again without noticing Sue in the crowd.

Did I tell Sue the disaster we had barely dodged? No way. She and Bob will likely meet again, as coincidences occur often in medical practice. He is now officially retired, not just underemployed, so he could turn up at any time.

In the
**EXAMINING
ROOM**

Goofy about gonads

Medical secretaries have seen it all, so my own personal assistant realizes there must be a logical explanation for any ruckus in my examining room. She knows that I generally work quietly, yet on some occasions she may hear me yell instructions not once but several times while my patient howls with hysterical laughter.

Why do some men giggle and wiggle once the examination of their genitalia begins? This step is usually the last in the annual checkup as most physicians do it, and by then the patient and I are settled nicely into the usual medical routine. We are engaged in light chatter, and I'm completely innocent and unprepared for the desperate challenge ahead.

Even the most sensible and mature male may react in this unexpected way. No doubt the patient is apprehensive by this point, and if I'm astute I will detect a catch in his voice and a distinct change in his body language when I ask him to lift up his undershirt while lying down. During the general examination, he will usually permit inspection of the upper abdomen and cooperate when asked to take a deep breath, allowing me to check the liver and spleen.

The trouble begins when I head south of his equator – the navel – but I push on, eliciting giggles while checking the lower abdominal quadrants. This part of our anatomy almost never yields detectable pathology on palpation – a good thing, no doubt, because real resistance has begun on the table before me and I am faced with rather rigid muscles and a moving target.

When asked to pull his Jockey shorts down, this patient may balk, actually holding the waistband to prevent my access. That won't do for any responsible and busy physician, so I offer gentle words of reassurance to get the darn underwear down as he continues to writhe and giggle. Progress is slow. This silliness continues once the gonads are fully exposed to air, and the patient may actually try to defend his equipment by pushing my gloved hands away, just as a giggling child anticipates having his ribs tickled.

Though the patient will readily agree afterward that this examination is an important part of his checkup, it requires real dexterity and persistence on my part to find an opening, launch another assault, and slowly conclude things as he howls. One man went to the extreme of nestling and secluding his entire equipment between his tightly closed thighs when I turned around to get my gloves. Imagine my surprise on revisiting the field of battle to find him apparently totally and bloodlessly castrated. Not at all fooled by this deceit, I insisted that he spread his thighs and allow me access – which he did, but again by centimetres.

Success is inevitable, but it may require careful strategy and flanking operations. While the patient is distracted protecting his testes, I may check his penis, and so on. Ordinarily, this whole process takes about thirty seconds. With these difficult cases, five seconds must suffice.

If the patient thinks our curious ordeal is over, he is wrong: I still have to check him for inguinal hernias. Asking him to stand on the floor and cough provokes even more hilarity. He will do so, but in a bent-forward posture while cupping his genitals, though they have already passed inspection. My hand anywhere nearby elicits more writhing, but in a young man the internal rings must be checked, and by now he is ready to break my fingers. Gentle reassurance allows me to enter these openings with my pinky, and I will not leave until he makes an adequate cough or pushes me away.

Once the examination is over, such a patient may apologize for this ridiculous behaviour, and I graciously accept his sentiments while reserving my own uncharitable thoughts on the subject. My

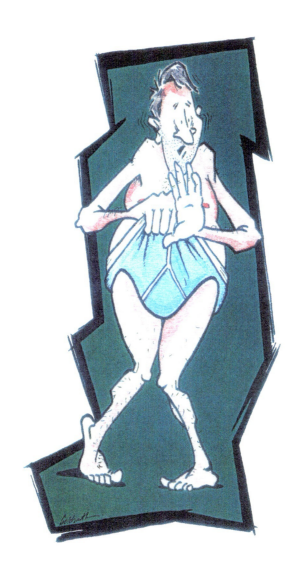

secretary gives me a funny look when I emerge from my examining room a few minutes later. She has heard the laughter, and some of these guys are still flushed and chuckling when they speak to her.

To prevent my being surprised again by such hypersensitive males at future visits, I always affix a large *G* on the outside of their files. This one letter identifies the guys who are goofy as far as their gonads are concerned.

The rear admiral

Every major hospital in Canada has a "rear admiral" in charge of delicate colorectal problems. In Edmonton my friend Dr. Donny Robinson had a favourite, who had helped many of his suffering patients. He finally had the misfortune to need this senior consultant's advice for himself, when his own anus became the central focus of his life.

Donny could no longer ignore this problem, as it had passed through stages A to H to X – the commonly known progression of Anusol to Preparation H to Xylocaine. All the pharmacies in Alberta could not help him. Even worse, he suspected that a recent need for antibiotics had created a dreaded problem that only a number 11 scalpel blade could cure: a thrombosed hemorrhoid. With the use of a mirror and some inspired contortions, the doctor saw the purple-tinged, tender globule that was tormenting him.

Donny looked forward with some trepidation to finally meeting the renowned surgeon in person. Shortly after they shook hands and spent a few seconds on the history, however, the admiral barked in military fashion, "Pants down and kneel here on my tilt table!"

Before Donny knew what was happening, his nose was six inches from the floor, and the surgeon was conversing with his bare butt. "Oh yes, looks like a juicy one. A bit of local anaesthetic and it's out. How did you get that?" Donny started to explain, but the exquisite pain of the infiltrating needle halted his speech. A few seconds more and he was cured.

Dr. Robinson could not express his thanks, as the admiral sailed ahead with his colonoscopy and began to talk about the medical profession and the weather. Amid flatus and suctioning sounds, they schmoozed on, as the physician submarined cautiously through Donny's tortuous innards. After a few minutes, the admiral told Donny's butt that he was all clear, and then he mercifully withdrew his periscope. Donny moaned in relief from the floor, where his head rested among the dust-bunnies.

The doctor helped Donny up, as he felt a bit seasick from the procedure, and said goodbye. He handed him some written advice about anal hygiene and proper maintenance. Donny still felt a bit woozy, so even after this close encounter he didn't know exactly what this physician looked like. He seemed amiable enough, though, from the chatter Donny had heard.

One of Donny's elderly patients had told him what to expect from this navy man during the procedure, and he was right on. The only conversation this patient could remember was "I like your shoes" – an appropriate comment considering their relative positions at the time.

Once the admiral had reassured him about his stern, Donny stepped briskly into the sunshine, happy in the knowledge of his restored health. He jauntily returned to his own practice, buoyed by the eager anticipation of talking to the front ends of his own patients and actually seeing their faces.

The window washer and the pelvic exam

Every young physician is amazed when coincidences occur in medical practice, but eventually we come to accept our unnatural powers. This phenomenon even has a name: synchronicity. The other day three factors came into play, leading to great embarrassment and apologies.

The medical building in which I work has five floors and about fifty narrow windows per floor. Window washers appear every six months, and we are warned several days in advance so we can protect our patients' privacy. In my practice, which is now largely geriatrics, I seldom do pelvic exams.

How was it possible that the window washer was standing on his scaffold smiling at me through the sheer curtains just when Mrs. J. Doe was about to have her pelvic exam?

By reflex I smiled and waved at him, to the surprise of my patient, whose business-end was fortunately directed away from the window. She said, "Who in the world are you waving at?" I hustled over to the window to pull down the blind. After my apology, once the examination was completed, we shared a nervous laugh. No doubt the inadvertent peeping tom shared his story with his buddies later that day.

Belly laughs

Medical offices are usually sombre places, quiet centres of healing where loud noise is most unusual. The patients in my waiting room were therefore surprised, then alarmed, by the loud peals of laughter coming from my office. At first, eyebrows were raised, but then they began whispering to each other. Was their physician practising a form of "primal scream" therapy? After ten minutes, the boldest of them approached my secretary to find out what was happening.

But she was just as puzzled. She knew that I normally worked quietly with patients – a nod here, a grunt of agreement there, and a soft conversational tone at all times. She also knew that I discouraged loud laughter among staff in the office, feeling that some patients might think we were having fun at their expense. To compound her puzzlement, she remembered that I was in my examining room with cranky Lotty, an elderly misery whose visits I dreaded. She was the howler.

To be professional, I should have stopped this unusual disturbance, but I wilfully kept it going. I had never seen this aspect of Lotty before, and I wanted to see how far she would go with it. Consequently, I let her hilarity roll on in waves, until she was flushed and sweaty and could hardly breathe. Can someone die from laughing so much? In part, my efforts were retaliation for her previous behaviour. In just one year as my patient, she had proved to be very peevish and opposed to most of my suggestions. She was also somewhat disrespectful to me and my staff.

The breakthrough with Lotty came as I was checking her bag full of medications. I innocently told her that I never reach into any such bag, as I have been surprised to find leftover food, knitting, or stool and urine samples there. For some reason, that remark touched her funny bone. In between her bellows, as she caught her breath, she said: "That serves you right, you know. You should trust your patients to bring in a list of their medications. The bottles are really not necessary." Hands on hips, while balancing precariously on my examining table, her body shook and heaved. I stood near lest she fall off.

When Lotty's laughter slowed down a bit, I mischievously added, "I have even found last week's socks and underwear in these bags." I watched in amazement as Lotty nearly screamed while laughing, making the windows rattle and the door vibrate. At this point my concerned secretary beeped me on the intercom to ask if I was all right. Not fully believing me, she knocked on my door and opened it, only to find me at Lotty's side, taking notes. By then, the patients in my waiting room had joined in with the infectious merriment and were having a great time of it, as strangers became friends.

The secretarial staff of the nearby offices had come over to see what was happening, accompanied by several dermatologists and gynecologists and one very skeptical psychiatrist. They also had a few chuckles and left shaking their heads.

Looking back, I now recall when I last heard such insane belly laughs – memories that might explain my perverse role in this episode. As a child, my parents took me to the Canadian National Exhibition, the large annual fair in Toronto. In the Midway, between the Freak Show and the House of Horrors, was a booth in which an enormously fat mechanical woman sat, laughing and rolling around continuously in this manner.

There were usually several rubes gawking at her and laughing along, soon to be enticed into her "Hall of Mirrors," where they too could appear four feet wide and ten feet tall. Several hours later, as we left the grounds, we still heard the fat lady laughing. Lotty put on the same kind of performance that day.

At last, I had found a way to disarm Lotty and make her lighten up. My only concern was whether I could make her stop. If not, there might be a job for her at the CNE.

Punmeister

My new patient appeared to be bad news. I watched as Ben, a boisterous gentleman in my waiting room, spoke to my receptionist. He then fixed his gaze on me, and we sized each other up, as strangers will. I passed muster, even though I was in the middle of a busy office day and rather flustered, but my white lab coat provided the camouflage I needed. His attire was a gaudy mix of grey suit pants, held up just below the nipples by a worn-out belt, and a multicoloured jacket – standard attire for male octogenarians in my practice.

My waiting room was jammed with patients, but Ben was not to be denied. He strode over and shook my hand a bit too firmly, asking, "Is this my new doctor?" I felt doomed. I was already half an hour behind, so that meant he would be kept waiting long enough to do serious damage to my other patients around him.

Like most physicians, I usually get a nice tingle of anticipation when faced with new patients. Most often they are the family members or friends of satisfied long-term patients, primed to expect good treatment. In turn, most physicians will try to make a good impression on the first visit.

Some of my colleagues screen potential new patients by telephone, but I generally let things take their course. My secretaries sometimes discourage callers, but I trust them to recognize psychopaths or doctor shoppers. To me, the only way patients and physicians can assess each other is face to face – and sometimes that leaves me vulnerable to surprises. Ben surely filled that role.

Ben had done his preliminary work over the phone well, asking my secretary about our favourite pastries. When I first laid eyes on him, he was doing something no patient had ever done before an initial appointment. He presented us with sweet treats from the local bakery for our break. Although this gesture sounds thoughtful and harmless, it's not necessarily so. I have sometimes tossed out gifts of food from disturbed individuals, and this time too I withheld judgment.

By the time I called his name, Ben was still quite feisty. He told me he was a retired entrepreneur and enjoyed working part time in his son's business because he loved kibitzing with customers. Predictably, he asked me to call him by his first name, but when I told him that was not my practice, he respected my habits. Anyone more than five years my senior, I explained, gets the respect I always offer such old-timers – and that is "Mr.," "Mrs.," or "Ms." before their surnames.

At that point Ben unleashed a torrent of puns. They were fun briefly but soon became an obstacle to history taking and the physical examination. When I said "anti-inflammatory," he said "uncle-inflammatory." When checking his chest I said, "Hold your breath," and he responded, "Where do you want it, in my hands or in a cup?" Enough said.

This hilarity had to stop, so I pressed on diligently but to no avail. Ben kept quiet only when he had a tongue depressor in his mouth, even gabbing during the sacrosanct ritual of measuring blood pressure. Perhaps he saw that I was getting less amused by his witticisms, so he briefly switched his patter to telling lengthy jokes. They were all clean and funny, and when he saw my smile and heard my laugh, Ben knew we were a good match.

During Ben's follow-up visit, I regained control of the field, telling him to cool it and threatening to silence him with a few more tongue depressors. We now get along fine: Ben provides a happy breather for us all in a business that has its serious side. Perhaps my neurologist colleague said it best when he described Ben, who was also one of his patients, as an "eighty-three-year-old George Burns clone." His urologist, who has since retired, actually audiotaped one of his visits.

When Ben comes next, I too will record his quips on a tape. He truly is a very humorous person. Flattered at this prospect, he has promised to bring along his best jokes for that occasion. And yes, we do eat his treats.

Emergencies – firefighters, police officers, and ambulance attendants

John at forty-nine had enough cardiac risk factors to gladden a team of physicians and lifestyle advocates. Personally, though, I had nearly given up on this reprobate. He could have used a personal trainer to get himself moving, a dietician to get him off fats, and several of the pharmaceutical industry's best products to control his blood pressure and diabetes and to eliminate his smoking habit. He was pre-coronary with his first step every morning, yet he carried on his career as an auto-mechanic and was the head of a happy household. Then at ten o'clock one Wednesday morning he developed chest pain while working under an Audi. A half-hour later he presented unannounced in my office, sweaty and pale.

My secretary informed me of John's arrival and sickly status, and within a few minutes, despite a normal ECG, we knew that his low blood pressure and the heaviness in his chest required a call to 911. As I held his hand, we heard the sirens blaring outside and, right after, two firefighters appeared at our door.

It's logical to ask why we needed firefighters. The older of these guys explained that normal routine in Toronto meant that they were the first of the three sets of responders to answer an emergency call. I outlined my patient's status to them but was told, "No, we can't take John to hospital. Our job is to resuscitate him if necessary." John, on seeing their oxygen tanks and other paraphernalia, seemed to improve. I agreed we could forgo the oxygen.

More sirens blaring outside announced the arrival of two paramedics pushing a gurney. Most emergency personnel arrive expecting the worst – and with this team you could see it in their nervous eyes. They looked as though they needed my help more than John did – as he appeared more comfortable by the minute.

He listened as I told his story again. Then a policeman entered the room, anxious to know what was going on. At this point John's distress level returned.

Next came the usual negotiations over whether the gurney in the waiting room should be brought into the examining room – a difficult job with our narrow corridors and door frames, already scratched and dented from previous assaults. I charmed the paramedics as the firefighters agreed John could walk the short distance to the waiting room.

There remained but one problem – John said he now felt fine and didn't want any further help.

By this time it was noon. Our staff were leaving for lunch, and John followed them out, passing unnoticed by the dozen other patients who by then had gathered to watch the proceedings. Out went the police officer, out went the paramedics pushing an empty gurney, and out went the firefighters.

Only after I had dealt with the many unhappy patients still waiting to be seen after his stealthy exit did I begin to feel less annoyed with John. Missing my golf date that Wednesday afternoon didn't help either.

Later, I learned that John had arrived at our local emergency department on his own. It seems he was somewhat sensitive about police officers. I found out in his Coronary Unit cubicle next day that not only had he failed to pay several parking and speeding tickets but that his driver's licence had been cancelled too.

My secretary's take on this overly crowded episode with rescue personnel all around? "Hey, they are all studs. What could be bad?"

Lying in state in the doctor's office

There are certain situations that are one-offs in a long medical career, or so I thought. How else to explain, on not one but two occasions, a body lying in state in the middle of my examining-room floor? Both times they were resting quite comfortably supine, arms across their chests, waiting patiently for my next move. Fortunately, their eyes were open and they were breathing.

Thirty years ago a recent immigrant, aged thirty-five, was having a checkup, and we had reached the point of "Please lie down." As I turned around to get my stethoscope, he made an unexpected move. I was shocked to see him lying on the floor, but I motioned to my examining table as a more suitable area for our next stage. He obliged.

Three decades passed before I saw this behaviour again, this time with a hale octogenarian. Again I had asked the patient to lie down and, before I knew it, he was smiling beatifically on the floor. He explained that he wanted to show me his prowess by getting up off the floor without help from me, and without grabbing my desk or my examination table for support.

I sensed that this performance was going to be really good, so I asked if I could call in my associate. We watched as he twisted and gyrated and huffed and puffed until he had righted himself. Looking at his watch, he announced a Guinness world record for eighty-five-year-olds of thirty seconds for his feat. He admitted he didn't have much competition in this sport.

That night I tried the same move. My wife walked into our living room and, thinking I was dead, shrieked. She was relieved when I rose up, and I am happy to say that I now hold the record in my age group for this manoeuvre – twenty seconds.

At my patient's next visit, with both of us lying supine on my waiting-room floor, I conceded him ten seconds as my secretary timed us. Then he beat me – but that could have been because other patients had arrived and I was a bit embarrassed by our horizontal hijinks.

The gamblers

The Province of Ontario used to outlaw all gambling except the Irish Sweepstakes. Then our leaders discovered how much money they could make if they ran casinos and allowed stores to sell lottery tickets. The rest is history.

On one occasion I looked into the waiting room and, for the first time in the fifteen years I had been treating him, saw miserable eighty-year-old Jack with a big smile on his face. When I called him in, I asked, "Why the smiles? Did you win the lottery?" "Yes," said Jack, "$100,000 in fact." We chatted a bit more about his winnings before I commented that now he could help out his kids. "No way," came his quick reply. "If I tell them, they will try to get it."

I don't bother with such things because I had a big win once and that was enough. A sweet elderly woman among my patients regularly bought a $1 lottery ticket for the folks looking after her, including her doctor and her hairdresser. When my ticket won $1,000, I was able to make a nice donation to my hospital.

I also have a bingo story and a casino story regarding my patients.

❖ ❖ ❖

Heaven must hold a special place for caregivers, and my sixty-year-old patient Mary will surely be twice rewarded at some point. Not only did she look after her very ill and very cranky eighty-five-year-old mother, who had kept her own apartment, but she also cared for her ninety-five-year-old disabled father-in-law, who lived with her and her own large family.

Mary somehow got Ma and Pa to a weekly bingo game, one of their few remaining pleasures, where a very dramatic part of this family saga took place. Mary told me one day that the caravan always entered the bingo hall the same way they entered my office. Before they even got through the door, other patrons heard them coming as Ma barked orders from her wheelchair as to which section of the sports arena she wanted to sit in. Her excitement and annoyance grew steadily, and she voiced it, commanding, "Mary, move faster, someone will get our spot. Don't be such a stupid idiot." As they progressed, Ma would clear a path through the crowd with her cane, spouting "Out of the way, out of the way, move it, coming through" at anyone blocking their path.

Once play started, Ma quieted down and ceased criticizing Mary, her nose into the four cards she was playing at the same time. But Mary knew that something was amiss when the caller announced, "Under the N, forty." It was a tradition in this bingo hall that all the players would loudly say "forty" if this number was called. On that occasion, however, Ma didn't call the number.

Mary took a close look at her mother from across the table. Eyes open, Ma seemed to be very slowly falling forward. When her chest hit the table, she stayed there, motionless. Mary grabbed her and shook her shoulders, with no response, so she screamed, "Call 911! I think my mother is ill."

Bingo players are very intent on the game. They tolerated this disturbance and paused only briefly as Mary raced around the long table to Ma's side, where she found her cradled tenderly in Pa's bony arms. Soon an alert nurse playing the game nearby checked Ma's pulse, found she had none, and began CPR after laying Ma on the floor with Pa's help.

All this activity took less than a minute, but it was too long a delay for some players, who began to hoot and hiss. They wanted to finish the game. "Under the O, sixty-two," droned the caller. "Under the B, twelve."

As Ma was tended to by the nurse, whose own game card was being tended to by a neighbour, Pa and Mary stood by helplessly, wringing their hands. At the moment the ambulance drivers arrived, the game came to a surprising conclusion. An elderly man who had been sitting beside Ma finished her card for her by yelling "Bingo!" Ma had won $400. She certainly would have died happier if her arteries had lasted just another five minutes.

Mary and her husband are still my patients fourteen years later, by now enjoying their own senior years.

◆ ◆ ◆

Blackjack, craps, roulette, baccarat, slot machines – you name it, casinos have it, and many of my patients have played there. No one has become instantly rich so far, but one patient may do well at great cost to her health. Here is a tale of greed and avarice, injury and assault, youth and old age. It does not have a happy beginning or ending. Rather, it is a sad comment on the social results of government-sponsored gambling casinos and the lust for gold they create among honest Canadians.

In the practice of medicine, we are constantly surprised by the stories brought to us by patients, and I was amazed to see eighty-five-year-old Jane limp slowly into my office one Monday morning after her day of debauchery. Her face was badly bruised, her arm was in a sling, and her spry step had become a limp, even though she was leaning on two canes. She was flushed with a high fever. As I examined her carefully, I saw many other bruises under her out-of-date clothing. Worst of all, she had fractured her coccyx, and her fever came from a urinary infection.

"Jane, dear Jane, what happened to you in that casino?" I asked, noting a shiner over this lovely little lady's eye. "Well, doc, it started this way," she began. "You know I belong to a club for seniors. Somebody came by and offered us a free bus trip to Orillia so we could win some money by gambling. He said all we had to do was sign up for the short trip – and off we went a week later."

Seeing my skeptical countenance, Jane continued, "Now doc, don't think I'm a foolish old lady. I've been around long enough to know what's going on in the world, and I fully intended to have fun and win. I brought $10 with me, and I was prepared to lose it all if necessary." I digested that bit about Jane's $10 limit and wondered who was in charge of these "free" trips. How could they take folks like her on such an excursion?

Jane continued after wincing when I palpated her fractured coccyx, then her flanks, eliciting signs of her kidney infection. "Doc, I spent twenty minutes in that casino blowing my ten bucks and nearly choking to death on the cigarette smoke. I had to get outside and look for a chair to sit on. I spotted a chair and plopped down, but it was on rollers, so over I went onto the concrete, pulling a desk down on top of me."

Imagining the commotion that followed as casino staff ran out to help her, I said to Jane, "That explains your bruises and broken tailbone, but how did you get a kidney infection out of this deal?" Embarrassed, she told me that the shock and the injuries had made her incontinent for a few hours, and she had endured a period wearing wet pants before the return trip.

In the following weeks, Jane saw her lawyer as well as me. He told her that the casino might be responsible for her mishap, and, if so, her $10 loss at one of the slot machines might turn a handsome profit from the casino's insurance company.

After a few weeks, everything but Jane's pride had healed, but she wondered if, at her age, she would be around for the resolution of her case. Perhaps casino staff will be more careful in future in choosing which people to invite along on their free trips. One guideline might be to avoid feeble and brittle-boned octogenarians – especially those with limited bankrolls and a $10 limit. But not so. I hear that the casino even picks up folks from nursing homes.

Two of my other elderly patients each sustained back and rib injuries in a casino while waiting for a slot machine to come free.

One lady finally noticed an empty machine, but the intense young woman beside it told her she was saving it for someone else. When the older woman moved in anyway, she was thrown to the ground, and her assailant fled. Another day a different patient was shoved against a machine by an overzealous waiter who jostled her.

These last two ladies continued to visit the casino regularly and have become members of the VIP Club. Apparently, if you throw enough money at the casino or visit frequently, management will provide private rooms, valet parking, and free meals. If you are particularly popular, they will even provide a hotel room at a reduced rate so you can stay closer to the action.

I also heard of a Toronto bank employee who embezzled money to feed his weekend habit. He was so popular in Las Vegas that a casino sent a limousine every Friday to pick him up after work and drive him to the airport. They paid for his airfare as well – until a bank audit discovered his crime.

At one of Jane's many follow-up visits for her injuries, she told me that the casino's insurance company had settled with her for $12,000. But before she received the cheque, she passed away, and her grandchildren have no doubt already spent it – not at the same casino, I hope.

ABOMINATIONS
and
EMBARRASSING
SITUATIONS

How to make your physician remember you

Some patients make life difficult for us physicians – even the most alert and experienced doctor may be defenceless against them. My "how-to" list for daring or mischievous patients is in no way comprehensive, as surprises occur daily in those little examination rooms where the unique doctor-patient relationship plays itself out. The physician may appear to hold the power, but some patients are dreaded if not feared. My quick list includes these items, set out here in alphabetical order. We all get our fifteen minutes of fame: make yours count if they take place in a physician's office. Doctors have long memories, so believe me, you will be remembered.

BARF: If you have stomach flu or the morning sickness of pregnancy, save some for the visit. Don't warn the doctor that you're feeling queasy because, if he has warning, he will have a basin ready. Try to miss that basin.

BELLY BUTTON LINT: Leave it untouched – any doctor will find this little accumulation impossible to ignore. Pretend to be unaware of it and ask to take it home after the doc removes it with tweezers.

BO: Surprisingly, body odour is not a common problem because most people are careful about personal hygiene. The sign that you really smell bad is the audible spray of room freshener as soon as you leave the examining room. Repeat offenders will detect signs of air freshener before they enter the room or even during the visit.

BROWN BAGS AND BOTTLE CAPS: Patients are constantly reminded to bring all their drugs to each visit, so toss them in a bag. Smile cooperatively as you hand it over, having first booby-trapped the bag with stool or urine samples, food and drink, news clippings, nail clippings, or even a change of underwear. Switch your tablets and capsules into the wrong bottles, then play dumb when asked to identify them. Leave some bottles poorly capped: you can literally bring your doctor to his knees as you both search valiantly for the pills spread out on the broadloom.

BURPS: These little belches may be excusable with some upper gastrointestinal problems, and eating onions before the visit will turn them into foul eructations. Some patients literally burp their way through a visit, particularly if they are asked first to lie down and then to sit up quickly again. They may erupt in so staccato-like a way that they can't even excuse themselves.

CLOTHING: Both genders at times may be wearing relics that make physical examination frustrating or even impossible. For women, I suggest full body girdles, enclosing the body from neck to crotch in a thick lining that an arrow could not penetrate. For a man, wear suspenders, which make the chest inaccessible, and in winter wear "combinations" – full-length one-piece underwear, neck to ankle, with a trapdoor hole in the rear for elimination. This garb will puzzle the doc, who doesn't know where to begin his examination. Outer clothing smelling of mothballs is another winner in spring and fall. One man discovered he could get more use out of the mothballs in his closet by putting them directly into all available pockets. I could smell him coming as soon as he got off the elevator on my floor.

COUGHS: These barks are expected in patients with colds, but when exaggerated, a cough can clear a waiting room pronto. Do not cover your mouth while hacking in the examination room, and let the doc have some phlegm at point-blank range when he checks your throat. Remember that doctors are fine actors, and their facial expressions may not show any discomfort. The evidence for a direct hit is written on their eyeglasses, if they wear them, or elsewhere on their faces and clothing. More experienced docs learn "the tongue-depressor dance" and are ready to lunge away as soon as the depressor reaches the back of the tongue.

FLATUS: If you are elderly or have intestinal problems, you may get away with passing wind. The doctor cannot move very far away because of the confined space. A special point to the hearing-impaired: just because you can't hear a toot doesn't mean the doc can't hear it, so a "silent-but-deadly" may be quite audible. The best part is that your polite doctor will ignore the noise and try not to wince once the smell hits home. Let's be honest here. Doctors get gas too, and I have sometimes taken advantage of a patient's deafness.

HANDSHAKES: When you are suffering from a cold and are covered with germs, insist that the doc shakes your hand on arrival, after the examination, and especially after he washes his hands. Only a brave doc can refuse an outstretched hand.

POWDER: For women, use copious powder under the breasts. Patients of both genders, arrive with liberal amounts of foot powder between your toes. That powder will stay in the doc's broadloom for weeks unless it is vacuumed up immediately.

SCENT: For women, wear strong perfume, as your healer's eyes may soon sting and weep. For men, slap on the aftershave lotion or cologne for the same result. As the doc reels from the reek, you may notice him staggering over to the door and opening it a bit or spraying the air freshener. Once I asked a woman not to wear perfume, saying I am allergic to scents, but it took me more than ten years of suffering to summon the courage to tell this lie.

SMOOCHES: If satisfied with the visit, show it by planting a huge kiss on the doctor's cheek or forehead, smearing him with lipstick. Don't let him refuse, even if he shows obvious revulsion and tries to escape. Younger women are forbidden to take this advice, as the doc might enjoy the embrace and get into real trouble. Male patients might kiss the doctor's hand, adding to his god complex. Doctors are wise to all these ploys and know that even the most adoring patients will switch loyalties the first time they call and can't get a convenient appointment.

SPIT: Patients who spit while they talk are one of a doctor's worst trials. If you are such a spitter, and if you have to come close because of poor hearing, congratulations – you win first prize. There is no defence except goggles and a face mask, so the healer must accept the saliva from six inches away. One lady deflects the evil-eye by doing *p-too, p-too, p-too* directly at me. Others spare me by doing the more customary *poo, poo, poo,* which can be said without being spread.

URINE: Bring it in whichever bottle is close at hand, in a sodden brown-paper bag that shows the leakage. For dramatic

How to make your physician remember you

effect, use a large yoghurt container with a wax-paper lid and slosh it over to the doc. No lid at all is even better.

WAX: When the doc syringes your ears, insist on looking at the disgusting contents of his basin. Watch carefully here, as wax and warm water sometimes fly out of your ear and may spray the doc's face and glasses. The doctor may try to hide the awful occurrence, but if it happens, say with a smile, "Did you get some on you?" Book your appointment just before lunch, knowing that your physician may prefer to skip food after such a visit.

How to make your patients remember you

We all have days when once-in-a-career accidents happen. In most cases the first incident is the one you learn from. If it happens again, you are basically an idiot. Here are some of my mishaps.

Things that wind up on the floor

Mishandling a poorly capped medication bottle will send scores of costly tablets or capsules to the floor, resulting in apologies and several minutes spent on your knees retrieving them. Then the decision whether to toss them in the garbage must be faced.

When preparing to give an injection of a medication costing $1,500, do not drop it. It will not be contaminated if you clean it carefully, but it doesn't look professional. After dropping a few tongue depressors on the floor, make sure the patient notices that you are using a fresh tongue depressor when you ask her to say "Ah."

Clear the floor of purses, bags, canes, and shoes around the patient before approaching. It is unseemly to stumble and stomp on a patient's gouty toe or to break someone's limb, including your own. The best place for a cane is the doorknob: you won't trip on it, it can't be forgotten, and the patient is disarmed – a consideration as your patients age and become demented and sometimes aggressive.

Noxious body products

While retrieving a urine sample from a high shelf, you must not absentmindedly tip the cup, resulting in a smelly spill on your clothing or the counter. Dip-sticking the floor or counter with a patient watching doesn't help. This wasted sample may have been produced after a prodigious effort from a prostate sufferer or anyone retention-bound with a bashful bladder. Never drink apple juice in the same place you test urine samples, for obvious reasons.

Ear syringing if done too forcefully can result in wax and warm water all over your face and clothes. I recommend goggles for this mess, as regular eyeglasses do not suffice. Do not register disgust when the bearer of a recurrent build-up of monstrous ear wax asks at every visit to check his ears. Try not to book his next appointment before your lunch. Resist the urge to triumphantly display a clump of belly button lint once you have released it from the unknowing patient with an "inny" belly button. Just toss it without comment.

Oops, I misspoke

Asking a patient how her spouse is doing is bad form if said spouse, your former patient, has died. When asking a buxom female patient to take some nice big breaths, do not ask her to take "nice big breasts." Listening carefully to what the patient is saying is wise before automatically mumbling "Good ... good ... good": she might be telling you someone has recently died.

Wardrobe malfunctions

A white lab coat covers many sartorial sins, but not if your trousers fall down all the way to the floor. In my case, this mishap could be blamed on my wearing low-slung jeans and forgetting to wear a belt. I hope the patient did not notice that I was trying to retrieve my pants while standing up to examine her.

It is fairly common for part of your lab coat to get caught on a doorknob as you whiz by or on the arms of your chair. After you have jerked to an unexpected halt, try to maintain dignity as you extricate yourself from the fix. If you can't, buzz your secretary for help.

Miscellaneous

Stabbing yourself while preparing or giving an injection is bad form, especially if you do so after injecting the patient, guaranteeing that you now share her problems too. Modern syringes are supposed to be idiot-proof. Guess what? They aren't.

UNCONTROLLABLE ACTS: If you get hiccups, take a drink and a break and clear the hiccups before seeing the next patient, who may brand you unfairly as a drunk. It is impossible to practise medicine while hiccupping.

SLEEPING ON THE JOB: Patients will accept a suppressed yawn or two, blaming it on a disturbed night. Once in a while someone might ask, "Are you getting enough sleep, doc?" They may even accept a brief nodding off for a few seconds, unless you forget what you were talking about and spout gibberish when you wake. Falling out of your chair sends a clear message that something is very wrong in the examining room.

TOOLS of the TRADE

Doctors causing high blood pressure

A war of nerves often takes place in my office between a patient and me. It features my stubborn streak and survival instincts against the patient's anxiety and impatience. Before the confrontation ends, we may both be rattled and in a sweat, with my salvation coming in my favourite numbers, 130/80. Oddly enough, this problem involves the routine testing of blood pressure (BP).

Primary-care physicians know that BP must be tested at every adult's visit or the patient will feel cheated. We learn early on that if we forget to measure BP, patients will ask for it just before leaving the room. Worse, they may remember it once they are in the down elevator and come back.

The act of taking blood pressure is a momentous ritual, supposedly done in silence and after the patient rests for several minutes alone in a separate room. These ideal conditions are difficult to achieve in a typical family practice like mine, which can best be described as a zoo. Ringing phones, babies crying, and an assembly line of patients coming and going are all part of this milieu, as is my desire to chat even while checking BP.

After silence is imposed, the game begins. Many patients stare intently at my face during the pumping up and releasing of the cuff's bladder, desperately analyzing my facial expression. While I may be daydreaming or thinking about lunch, their spirits rise or fall with each twitch of my nose or lift of my eyebrow. Every pensive pose can dash a patient's hopes, while every hum, as I sing along to the music in my head, can send the viewer's spirits soaring. What power we docs have!

Their eyes move from my face to the BP cuff itself, squinting at the highest numbers reached as the systolic reading is overshot.

They nearly faint when the numbers reach the 200 mark, unaware that this temporary figure means nothing at all. They stagger from the implications, sure of their imminent demise. All this worry only makes the pressure go even higher.

My reveries cease when patients want to know their blood-pressure readings, especially if I have not been playing close attention. Subconsciously I know that the numbers fall in the normal range, but some inquisitive people create a dilemma by insisting on knowing the actual figures. If such patients have never had a problem, I fib and tell them that the reading is 130/80. Most are happy with that.

Hypertensive patients are more demanding because they know their usual BPs and will not be satisfied with 130/80. With them, I stall for time and create some additional unease by saying, "I will tell you the reading after I do the other arm." I pay closer attention this time, and they are relieved with the good news, actually sighing in relief.

BP can be very difficult to hear, sometimes requiring several efforts. This delay is troubling for the patients and frustrating for the physician. I regularly start on the left arm, in the sitting and the standing positions, but these two steps are divided at times by patients asking, even pleading, to know the reading.

The field of play is again moved to the other arm, after I refuse to give them the first results, having been burned many times and forced to eat my words when the numbers on the other arm differ greatly. At this point, the more neurotic become downcast and respond, "It must be high – I can tell." I maintain silence and show no mercy. Tension builds between us over these several minutes as I check the other arm's pressure – dissipated only with my belated exhalation of 130/80 or numbers close to those.

Far worse are patients whose BP cannot be heard at all, devils whose arteries lie deep enough to defy detection. A confession: if I cannot detect any sound after a few minutes, the patient is dismissed with 130/80 and my hope for better luck at an early follow-up appointment. I must also confess that sometimes the patient and I are not even sure if I have in fact measured the BP. It is done so slickly and routinely that it can disappear as we converse. Those little pressure lines left on the biceps prove that I did the BP, and I close the topic again with my favourite numbers.

It has been shown that doctors inadvertently raise BP through "white-coat syndrome." In my experience, this reaction adds 10–20 points to the reading, or 50 points if I am nasty and having a bad day – and the patients know it. Thus I plead with patients to buy a BP monitor and test themselves at home, where they are relaxed. Because these home readings are always lower and generally quite accurate, this personal responsibility can prevent decades of unnecessary overtreatment. At times drugs can be discontinued if the patient home monitors BP after stopping a drug.

Finally, a piece of advice for forgetful or distracted colleagues: remember to put the earpieces in your ears. There can be no face-saving 130/80 if the patient spots the stethoscope still hanging around your neck and asks, "Doc, aren't you supposed to be listening with those things?"

The stethoscope – the colder the better

A very embarrassing thing happened to one of my fellow medical students early in our training. He was asked to listen to a patient's heart and to give us a description of the heart murmur he was hearing. He did so admirably, not realizing that his stethoscope was not plugged into his ears. The staff man kindly pointed this omission out, and my friend later became a cardiologist – perhaps for this reason.

The stethoscope remains invaluable for diagnosing respiratory infections, emphysema, and asthma, as well as heart murmurs and arrhythmias. It is part of every examination for adult patients and is usually used to check blood pressure. Its use is now centuries old, but it remains vital and is the first step, even in this age of echocardiograms and a multitude of other cardiac tests. A good set of ears is required, and cardiologists are said to be better able to ascertain weak heart sounds and murmurs. Still, it must be the family physician's ears that get the ball rolling, leading on if necessary to tests and consultations.

What is less known is that stethoscopes can carry germs if they are not cleaned between patients. It joins unwashed hands, dangling ties, loose long sleeves, and door handles as purveyors of bacteria. My guess is that some stethoscopes have not been cleaned since 1980. A simple cotton ball in alcohol swabbed across the diaphragm will do the job just fine.

Any physician who treats small children knows that they like to yank the stethoscope out of our ears, and it can give us a nasty whack in the face if we are careless when removing it. Some patients may wonder why we wear it draped around our shoulders rather than our necks when not in use. The reason is simple: if it is tight around the neck it may reduce circulation to the brain, and that is generally considered a bad thing.

I am sure that some doctors have used a stethoscope against certain patients as a weapon – simply by not warming it up. This application works especially well when making house calls in the depths of a Canadian winter. It also decreases the chances of future demands for unnecessary house calls – as I know all too well from experience.

The many uses of the humble tongue depressor

My very capable secretary once misread an ad for tongue depressors – and a suitcase filled with them was delivered to our door. After my associate and I stopped laughing, we considered shipping them back or donating them to our hospital. Instead, we kept them and looked forward to decades without another purchase. All that happened, however, was that we became very profligate and imaginative about their use.

During lulls in my office schedule, it became great fun to take out my bottle of glue and create a thicket of stars and stripes or a farmhouse with a corral for horses. The possibilities were endless once I bought a child's painting kit. At this point I had to hide my enjoyment, as my secretary began rolling her eyes.

I discovered how to make a weapon that could propel a large calcium tablet with great force at the backside of unpopular departing patients, but I got too accurate and hit Mrs. Jones on her ample butt. When she yelped and turned around, I quickly hid my ammunition and played the innocent. The white powder was the only sign on her clothing after the tablet smashed on impact. My walls were also a mess. After that experience, I practised only on the departing rumps of male drug reps.

Tongue depressors also make satisfactory shoehorns in a pinch and can be used as Popsicle sticks to create healthy orange-juice snacks in my freezer. Because I am always doing minor carpentry repairs around the office, I have found them to be excellent shims when projects demand levelling.

The result? The suitcase was empty in just four years.

Throat examinations are largely useless rituals in general medical practice, except for throat infections. Even then, not much is seen to distinguish viral from bacterial infections. Still, the examination must be done, so I must dodge gag-spittle-spray boluses sent my way. Moreover, I often tell patients that I don't really need a tongue depressor to peruse their tonsils. My usual quip goes as follows: "You have such a big mouth, I won't need it." They seem to find this line amusing.

The nerd pocket

Dork or doofus, nerd or brown-noser – we all know this awkward type, and it's almost always a male. In public school he will be the teacher's pet, rewarded with such responsible jobs such as hall monitoring or blackboard duty. In high school he will be the serious guy with lots of time on his hands for study, though female companionship will generally be unattainable. High marks are usually the by-product.

When our overachiever enters university in a professional field such as medicine, success generally follows. It's often spectacular, as nature evens out the playing field in the end. His badge of honour is the "nerd pocket," found on the left of his plaid shirt or lab coat. While the sharp guys in high school wear pocketless polo shirts and keep their pens in their backpacks, the nerd's narrow chest fairly bristles with writing instruments and schedules, reminder lists and rulers.

This image came to my mind as I was extricating the tip of my tie from the K-basin containing warm water and a patient's just-removed soft earwax. It was not the first time this unpleasant accident happened or the first soiled tie I brought home to my wife.

There are two alternatives to preventing this disgusting cleaning problem: my old method was whipping my tie over my left shoulder before bending over a sink, but that's risky because the tie can flop down again. My new and improved method is tucking the tip of my tie deep into my nerd pocket until the danger of bending over is past. This solution is foolproof.

Without my nerd pocket I have no place to tuck the innumerable reminder notes that keep my life and my practice going – Mr. Smith's referrals and Mrs. Jones's legal letter do not get done, nor can I return phone calls. The twenty-dollar bill or cheque I received from a patient is not tucked away next to my heart but winds up loose in my pants' pocket, only to be forgotten and lost the next time I reach in for a tissue.

Worst of all, I have nothing to write with because all my pens have gravitated to one room among the several I use. I have to interrupt patient visits and wander in frustration from examining room to consulting room to secretary's station in search of a pen or pencil to record the history. I become quite unpopular with my secretaries and my associate when in desperation I swipe one of their pens.

The only disadvantage with my favourite storage department is the chance that I may well leave a cheque or a money note there, only to have it go through the washer and the dryer. A fine example of physician money-laundering!

PECULIAR PATIENTS

Doorknobs, handshakes, and other hazards

My wife has accused me of being obsessive-compulsive. I agree to some extent, but I finally met my match in a patient. Joe Brown, an elderly retired medical technician, was bad news in my waiting room. No other patients wanted to sit beside him – and if they did so without looking at him first, most soon moved away because of his manner and appearance.

His clothing was shabby, and he wore it in several layers at once. While not a street person, he always carried a large bag or a suitcase with a change of clothing and various oddities. I eventually found out why he needed extra clothing – as I explain below. He had a somewhat wild and worried look and could be aggressive. Once, when I called him into my office, another man named Peter stood up in error. Joe walked up very close to him and said loudly, "Is your name Joseph Brown?" Peter, a former paratrooper, told me he had been quite prepared to shove Joe to the floor if he touched him.

Once we were in the examining room, other problems became evident. His ancient underwear was torn in many places, and on occasion pieces fell off. I always had an irresistible urge to tidy up the floor of my examining room while still talking to him – and I did. Joe didn't mind – he even helped, amid his apologies. He actually apologized at least twenty times per visit. To complete this picture, Joe's copious amounts of foot powder soiled the broadloom in my examining room. After his socks and shoes were back on, we both sprang into action. I took a damp cloth to the footstool he had sullied while he vacuumed my carpet. None of this behaviour was strange to my staff: they equipped my examining room specially before his visits. They were happy not to be responsible for the cleaning themselves. And Joe sheepishly begged their pardon on his way out.

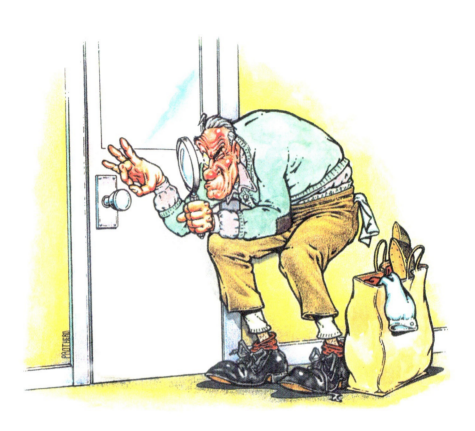

All physicians attract an assortment of medical groupies – patients who worship them – and Joe was one of mine. They constantly profess their devotion, but this adoration may become tiresome and possibly harmful as time goes by. With a beseeching face, Joe constantly repeated that he trusted my medical judgment "explicitly." He brought tributes of candy, popcorn, and other treats for me and my staff, despite my weak protests. At first I would not sample anything from Joe, but later I gave in to my sweet tooth. At my hospital, I bumped into his cardiologist. Yes, he too had received candy, but because he was skeptical about Joe, he gave it to his staff.

Joe saw nothing wrong with my own peculiar rituals, some of which are seasonal. Over the years he learned to assist me in picking up leaves from the floor in the spring and fall, and salt pieces tracked in from the streets in winter. Unlike other patients, he was not surprised every October when I chased and swatted flies. In fact, he drove them in my direction, letting me, like a safari hunter, make the kill. While other patients wondered why I was running around the room swinging a rolled-up journal, Joe knew instantly. Some patients thought this frenzy some kind of medical priestly spell, but others who didn't see well got a bit frightened at my exertions.

Early on, I noticed that after each visit, Joe would not handle any doorknob directly but would use a cloth or his shirt to wrap it first, apologizing all the while. He explained that all knobs in a doctor's office must be covered in germs. He did not want to catch any microbes, and he didn't want me to catch his variety either. He instructed me not to shake hands with patients, because I often don't know why the patient is visiting me. However, it's usually the most infectious patients who insist on a firm handshake.

Other difficulties flowing from this misguided hygiene were immediately obvious. I pointed out to Joe that my patients and I would be stuck in my examining room until each of us caught on and opened the door. And how would I ever bring myself to touch a patient at all? Joe apologized for confusing me. He then had other sage advice, which has not only helped me to avoid germs while still maintaining a measure of etiquette but also reduced the need to wash hands by 50 percent or more. In short, he advised me to use my left hand for turning doorknobs and greeting patients. It's easy to occupy the right hand by holding the chart – and a left-handed grasp is better than no handshake at all. In this way my pen, telephone, and other equipment stay cleaner, after being touched by only my right hand.

There is more. During one visit Joe said, "Look doc, I'm sorry to point this out, but you are continually licking your right middle finger while leafing through my file. Don't you see how much better it is to keep your right hand germ-free?" I could not argue with his logic and thanked him. The result? I seldom catch colds now.

The reason why Joe carried extra clothing with him finally became apparent much later, as he again proved his devotion to me. As luck would have it, the bank in my office building was robbed just before his appointment time, and the police prevented anyone from entering the building. Predictably, Joe caused a disturbance with the officers, who sent him away. To my surprise, he succeeded in getting to me by walking around the block, pulling out a different set of clothes from his bag, changing in an alley, and sliding past the police. Astonished, I asked Joe why he had bothered. He said he was like "an old thief," used to danger and capable of camouflage. Touchingly, he said he could not rest until he knew I was all right.

Joe's paranoia and compulsions stemmed from his youth in Europe, when events during the Second World War destroyed his world. Tragedy struck his young family several times later while he lived in the United States.

He went on to have coronary artery bypass surgery, which he breezed through. Predictably, when I visited him in hospital, some of the nurses on his floor had some interesting comments about his cleaning and apologizing routines. His overly generous supply of flowers and candies to each of them had softened their hearts, although most of them still left his room shaking their heads and smiling. Bacteria finally did get him when he developed acute leukemia, leaving him prone to infection. Pneumonia then claimed him after a brief struggle.

Examining-room ballet

When we have a full waiting room and people are getting restless, I ask my staff to call the next patient in. They see me first in my white lab coat, with a stethoscope draped around my neck. This guise establishes respect and confidence, and even on a bad-dress day the coat hides a lot of sins.

If the patient has been hacking up a lung or two in the waiting room, I maintain a four-foot "comfort zone," mandated by the dangers of potential contagion. For the same reason, I don't shake hands, but clutch the protective patient file against my chest. Both the patient and I wear masks.

We sit at opposite sides of my desk, have a brief chat, and get down to business. Off comes some clothing, followed by draping, and I direct the patient to climb aboard the examining table. I approach cautiously, say a little prayer, and hold my breath as I check heart and lungs while avoiding exhalations. The duration of this physical exam is determined by how long I can avoid breathing before turning blue. The older I get, the briefer this examination gets – certainly less than thirty seconds.

I hurry away as the patient dresses and keep both our hands busy with requisitions and prescriptions. Then the race is on to the doorknob: I lunge ahead, throw the door open, and dash out. If the patient gets to the doorknob first and contaminates it, my escape is blocked.

After his routine, the patient becomes my secretary's problem. She too is no slouch in this antimicrobial dance and almost always has a follow-up appointment card ready. Still masked, the patient is directed to leave, and he is given a wide berth by other patients.

The Typhoid Mary routine can also be used for patients with body odour, for women who bathe themselves in perfume, and for men who splash on too much cologne. The only modification is that I spray the room with air freshener before, after, and at times during the visit. I am no good to anybody if I pass out.

Fainters, grabbers, and smoochers

One attention-seeking lady fell exhausted into a chair immediately after signing in with my receptionist. Another one went much further, falling on the floor as soon as she showed her health card to my secretary. All we doctors have patients like these two, who could easily qualify as stage actors. My thespians were then about seventy years old. The episodes were very frightening for the other patients, who immediately rushed to the women's aid. Initially their behaviour brought me running to their sides at the expense of other patients. Later my reactions were decidedly mixed – and somewhat dramatic.

Sally was definitely an ill woman, but not as bad as she pretended. As she collapsed into the chair, she followed through with much moaning and gasping and fanning her face with her hands. It turned out to be her attempt to jump the queue. Eventually she stopped, after I began to ignore her. First, though, I had to explain my reasons to the patients gathered around her, who were attempting resuscitation. I will admit, however, that Sally was a fine performer, desperately difficult to disregard.

My associate and I often saw Sally looking quite fit in our local shopping plaza. She was almost athletic in her grace as she did her rounds. We never greeted her on these occasions because she's the sort of patient physicians try to avoid at all cost – by crossing the road and dodging cars if necessary.

Sally's case has a postscript: she was admitted to hospital in 2010, fifteen years after I first wrote this story, and was treated by a frustrated colleague. Not only did he agree with me about her but took a big chance and put his reservations in writing. He used the words "plaintive, importuning, disruptive, argumentative, non-compliant and abusive" in his discharge summary. He knew she was improved after two days in hospital, "given her ability to talk quite loudly and forcefully." She was strong enough to repeatedly visit the nursing station and "be even louder and more difficult," no doubt sending the more experienced staff away in a blind panic when she approached. I hoped that Sally or her family would never see his report, as it would raise many questions for my hospital's ombudsman.

My biggest mistake with Sally involved her progeny. With the passage of time, considering that she was much older than I was, I knew that eventually she would leave my office in peace. That proved to be true, but before she died she beseeched me to assume the medical care of her son. In a weak moment I accepted him as a patient. He turned out to be quite a character himself, but as yet, fortunately, he has not adopted her waiting-room tactics.

Nellie's problematic personality was described to me in advance by Les, an associate who was leaving his practice. Like a man relieved of a heavy weight, he put his arm around me and wished me luck while chuckling about this woman. I knew I was in big trouble when our staff joined him in a few hearty laughs.

At her first appointment with me, Nellie began with that awful phrase, "I am not a complainer, but ..." She produced several lists of diseases and drugs, then rattled off symptoms until my head swam. After the visit, she said she liked my style and promised eternal loyalty. Horrors! As time went by I could handle Nellie's demands until she added a new and unique routine. She did not like waiting her turn for my attention, so began collapsing on her arrival, conveniently in the corridor to my examining room. My heart hardened after a while. To end this charade, which was frightening to other patients, I simply let Nellie lie there until I was free. I then carefully stepped over her prostrate body and said, "Next please." That patient and I would then gingerly climb back over Nellie and go about our business. My behaviour disturbed other patients, but once I explained Nellie to them, they acquiesced in my program and let her lie there. After several more episodes, Nellie no longer tried this stunt.

I did have a stroke of good luck with a third patient, Mrs. Smith, my champion importuner, who grabbed my sleeve and held it firmly whenever we met, be it in the bakery, in the hospital, or in my office. She fired me for some reason, but "begged" to return a few months later. I had the satisfaction of refusing this request because of my new office policy, invented just for her: "No patient who leaves and transfers to another physician can come back to the practice." She's still trying, but I refuse to crack.

Finally, we come to a major problem. In a small examining room it is almost impossible to avoid patients who want to kiss my hand or my forehead or, worse, plant a kiss on my cheek, leaving lipstick until I can scrub it off. These big fans will be the first to switch doctors once they can't get a convenient appointment with me, so I dodge and weave until their passion fades.

The carrot people

John and Mabel smelled a bit strange when we shook hands on their first visit. Both in their sixties, they seemed like an ordinary couple, except that they both had orange complexions. It was summer, and they both wore short-sleeved shirts. I couldn't help but notice the vivid orange staining on their arms up to their elbows. As I began to take John's history, all the wheels in my head were searching for an answer to this odd colouration.

John had been referred to me by Doctor Smith, an assertive and feisty cardiologist, after an admission for a severe myocardial infarction with some heart failure. As my new patient handed me the consultant's letter of referral, he said I should ignore the recommendations just as he had done, dismissing them as so much wasted ink. His comments surprised me: I knew that Dr. Smith was a no-nonsense type with patients, and they commonly found his old-school manner quite intimidating. As for me, I quaked whenever he and I spoke about a mutual patient, even over the phone!

John had discarded his prescribed medications. Instead of the post-coronary routine of beta-blockers, digoxin, and blood thinners, he and his wife were following a carrot-regimen given them by a herbalist. Orange people were new to me, so I checked out "carotenemia" in my Merck Manual. Apparently it could progress to harmful "hypervitaminosis A" for people who ate polar bear or seal liver. But carrot crunchers like my duo were safe and were usually diagnosed by a discolouration of the skin, especially on the palms of their hands and the soles of their feet.

John and Mabel certainly had these features generally, but the excess forearm pigment came from mornings spent happily cleaning and peeling pounds of carrots and blending carrot juice. John stated boldly that he did not trust most physicians and their use of drugs, and he went on to say he had cancelled further cardiac tests and appointments with Dr. Smith. I listened patiently, thinking that this little man must have fried his brain during his infarction. Until then I was no advocate of herbal remedies for advanced heart disease.

I added John and Mabel to my list of oddball patients and wondered how long their luck would last. The answer came sixteen months later, with John's second heart attack. After two weeks of chest pain that the herbalist could not relieve, John came to my office, and I easily diagnosed the cause with an ECG. Only after much argument did he agree to go back to the hospital. There he engaged in a second battle of strong wills with Dr. Smith.

The medical resident sent me a note four days later when John signed himself out of hospital, without any investigation being done and no prescribed medications. "This patient is of the belief that we in the medical profession use patients for experiments, and that any drugs given would make him worse and kill him."

John did, quixotically, agree to see Dr. Smith in a follow-up examination two months later, and it was in Smith's hospital office that the decisive third battle was fought a few weeks later. Dr. Smith was furious, as was obvious in the consultation note he sent me. "I saw this super-stubborn patient ... who adamantly refuses any help, and therefore I see no point in wasting his or my time." Smoke seemed to rise from the printed page as Dr. Smith concluded, "I sincerely hope that Mother Nature will be kind to him." She was. John and wife are still doing well five years later, though he now has a pacemaker.

For readers who are interested, I will gladly forward some wonderful carrot recipes my patients have created for me. And if you're a doctor and you meet an orange-coloured smelly colleague at a conference, please say hello.

Whistlers and hummers

Some of my favourite older patients, all men, whistle softly and hum as they go through life. In my office, their pleasant harmonies may accompany history taking, doffing and donning clothes, and physical examinations. Imagine my surprise, then, when I felt threatened with knives by my most amiable hummer!

Whistlers and hummers establish rapport with me instantly because I sense I am in the presence of mellow individuals. They pause in their reveries only when they must pay strict attention to my instructions and advice. Then they whistle their way out to the waiting room, where their music and relaxed body language put others at ease. Mike was a seventy-five-year-old bachelor when he became my patient, referred to me by his widowed girlfriend, Mary, who was the same age. An artist, Mary had presented me with several beautiful watercolour miniatures over the years. But Mike was her biggest contribution to my life.

Their relationship became clearer to me by an oddity I discovered on Mike's first visit to me – something in his boxer shorts which I had never seen before. I detected a string around his neck, leading right down into his underwear, where it disappeared. My curiosity aroused, I followed its course and extracted a whistle.

This object demanded an explanation: Mike told me that he and Mary both carried whistles as locating devices in large department stores. She was concerned that, like most men, he would dawdle around these premises, while most women go straight into the practical business of browsing and buying.

When Mary needed Mike to try on a sweater or trousers, he was not available. Again like most men, he was lost among the displays of sporting goods, candies, or women's lingerie. Mary's solution was to blow her whistle loudly a few times (both were hearing impaired), just as a bird trills to find its mate. This method was foolproof for them: Mike followed these sounds and always appeared with a sheepish grin after about ten minutes.

Occasionally, Mike used his own whistle to locate Mary, when he got bored or lost. They both attracted stares and comments from sales staff and other shoppers, and Mike was once accused of treating his girlfriend "like a dog." The only question left to me about Mike's whistle was why he kept it in his shorts.

"Well, doc, you know, if I keep the whistle on my chest, it interferes with my suspenders," said Mike, "and if it rests around my midriff, it gets stuck in my belt." This explanation sounded reasonable to me. "And it tickles my fancy sometimes, if you get my drift," he added with a sly smile. Enough said. Although curious, I never asked him where Mary kept her whistle.

Now in his dotage at age eighty-five, Mike recently surprised me by bringing a vicious set of kitchen knives to a visit. Fortunately, they were not dangling in his Jockey shorts! I found them in a brown-paper bag as I looked for his medication bottles. I escaped injury because I have long ago learned not to reach into such bags, fearing what I might find there. As usual, I inverted his bag, producing a loud clang as the knives and a hatchet fell to the floor. Meanwhile this sweet and gentle man kept humming along. Still, I demanded an explanation.

It appeared that Mike and Mary were no longer love birds because he had become infatuated with the young woman who cuts his hair. "She is really nice to me, doc, and we spend a lot of time chatting as she trims my hair," said the nearly bald Mike. "My appointment with her is right after my appointment with you." He spoke of her in glowing terms and told me that the knives were intended for this woman as a "tip." His gift still bore the $5 price tag that had attracted him at a garage sale.

I was not sure whether this courtship was going anywhere. Mike told me, "We usually eat lunch together in the back of her shop," so something was going on. But the thought of Mike's barber sharpening up those blades for possible use on her clients made me wince – especially because I go to the same salon.

PHYSICIANS' BAD HABITS

Performing ritual Sudoku in medical practice

I have become addicted to Sudoku, that mathematical puzzle that appears in every newspaper. It has affected my professional life as a physician and much of my leisure time. My patients are not suffering, but that could change. In a way, my approach to Sudoku is similar to taking a health history from a patient.

There are eighty-one squares in Sudoku – just as there are often about eighty-one years in a person's life. Some squares represent health problems, poor lifestyle choices, and opportunities taken or missed. When new patients of various ages come to me, most of them have many of their squares filled in – just as every Sudoku has twenty-five or thirty of its squares already taken. I cannot affect the past in either case, but as a physician I can certainly try to affect the future.

A history of cancer found early and removed might use up just a few squares, while cancer misdiagnosed might use up most of the nine boxes, leaving me few options to improve my new patient's health and achieve a satisfactory conclusion. Over the many years of a patient's relationship with a family physician, a misstep early on by an inattentive physician or a frightened patient ends the game and the life prematurely.

We can reverse our steps with an eraser in Sudoku, but not so in life. There is absolutely no guesswork in Sudoku, and there should be none in medicine. In a big city, it is easy to investigate everyone with suspicious chest or abdominal pain or signs of a pending stroke or coronary. The list is endless, but guesswork, such as minimizing or ignoring a patient's symptoms, can be fatal.

Only a few of my patients are aware of my obsession with Sudoku, and they know about it only when I spot them puzzling over it in the waiting room. Once they enter my examining room, I confess my own fascination with the game, and we spend the first few minutes of the consultation passing tips to each other, before the business of medicine must grudgingly be commenced.

Sudoku is truly a ritual. Some do it against the clock or in competition, but these conditions seem a waste to me. To perform Sudoku, you must have time and patience in the face of what may seem impossible odds. The numbers 1 to 9, and only one of each, must be placed in each of nine intersecting rows, columns, or boxes.

The grunt work of performing Sudoku involves probing twenty-seven rows, columns, and boxes for possibilities, slowly eliminating numbers, and changing the game with every number dropped. I find that I can easily do one stage at a time between patients. The problem lies in the natural urge to follow up success immediately, damn the consequences.

My secretary knows what is going on when I close the examining-room door after a patient leaves, and she makes excuses on my behalf when things are delayed. Staff get concerned only when I fall far behind, but that's not generally a problem. The ominous rumble from the waiting room, known and feared by every physician, lets me know when the natives are restless and it's time to put the Sudoku down.

If I am really on a roll, I can actually perform Sudoku during the patient's visit. I simply scan it while the patient's back is turned away during chest examinations. Traversing the chest with my stethoscope, once I know that the chest is clear, I say, in time-honoured fashion, "Please take a few more deep breaths." There's always the danger that someone, impressed with my thoroughness, will continue taking big breaths until hyperventilated and fall off the table, but so far that has never happened.

My morning Sudoku ritual involves waking an hour early to prepare myself emotionally and to allow ample time for a leisurely beginning. When my *Globe and Mail* arrives at the office, I must resist the strong urge to tackle it immediately. Instead, I hustle over to the office photocopier, where I enlarge the Sudoku and make a few copies. Extra copies are needed because failures are common, especially with all the distractions of a medical practice.

Seated at my office desk, not expecting patients for some time, my ritual continues. When all is ready, I put pencil to paper gingerly. One false move ends the game prematurely: as it happens, that is a fairly good outcome, because finding out you have failed with only two or four of the eighty-one numbers to go causes extreme anger and frustration. I can't let sensitive patients see such emotions, so once I find myself off track, I toss the puzzle and immediately begin again with a different approach.

Early in my Sudoku studies, a good friend who is also a patient noticed a puzzle on my desk and gave me an excellent clue. It solved the problem, but I am no longer satisfied with easy puzzles. He meant well, but he created a monster.

Back home after a hard day performing Sudoku while seeing patients, exercise becomes difficult as well. Sudoku is clearly impossible while on my treadmill and barely doable on my Exercycle, because the delicate notations require a fine hand. However, in good weather you might spot me walking outside with a pencil and clipboard, head down and quite absorbed in Sudoku. My neighbours with whom I used to chat are surprised to hear me mumbling various number combinations and so absorbed that I barely say hello to them or their adorable babies and ugly dogs. They may interpret my behaviour as unfriendliness or worse. Can we label this new disease as "Sudoku psychopathy" – a manifestation of an obsessive-compulsive disorder?

Other activities have actually become somewhat easier. At medical conferences I sit at the back to perform Sudoku. The speakers don't recognize that I'm listening with only one ear and assume, instead, I'm madly writing down their every word. This new routine is an improvement for me, because my customary habit was to nod off. At my last meeting I remained somewhat attentive and conscious for the first five speakers, until my Sudoku was done. Content, I joined my few colleagues already deep into their slumbers.

With clipboard in hand, I can assist my wife in the local supermarket, wait in the car while she does some chores, and even go to a movie, armed with a small flashlight if the film is boring. Being with friends in restaurants or in someone's home provides further opportunities if I turn the conversation to Sudoku. Many friends are similarly smitten and willing to admit it; they help me out with the Sudoku that is always close to my heart in my nerd pocket. Others are willing to learn, and I have introduced them to my philosophy.

At funerals, I can appear to be quite solemn during the eulogies, while scribbling away quietly and dabbing my eyes. At the Rogers Centre for Blue Jays baseball games, a Sudoku is invaluable and can be hidden in the centre of the program. Religious services hold no fear for me now. A puzzle secreted in the holy literature keeps me alert and prevents me from embarrassing myself by falling asleep. Again, a seat at the rear makes most sense, lest my neighbours notice any sacrilegious activity.

For those interested, I suggest not starting Sudoku until you have consulted an expert, Sudoku.com, or a book on the subject. If you jump right in, you may face needless and endless frustration.

Finally, if you need help, ask a teenager or a child – in my case, a granddaughter.

The five-pound Hershey bar

There is no convenient way to approach John's giant Hershey bar. It is a foot wide, two feet long, and about three-quarters of an inch thick. If you put it in the fridge, you pretty well need a hammer and chisel to chop off a piece. My staff know what I'm doing because they hear the hammering and grumbling going on in my office behind closed doors and sometimes see chocolate smears on my lab coat and face after I have gnawed on it.

That I have finally reached the depth of substance abuse can be blamed on this five-pound solid chocolate bar John gives me every year for Christmas. He does so because he appreciates the house calls I make to his disabled elderly mother.

You see, I get all my chocolate free, thanks to subtly manipulating my patients. I feel like one of Pavlov's dogs when I examine my office schedule at the start of each day. Sweets make some of the most difficult patients tolerable when I remember their previous gifting habits. They may demand much more of my time than others at each visit, but I begin to salivate if I glance at the package in their hands. They are favoured even if they are sometimes empty-handed, on the same Pavlovian principle. On the completion of the visit, I exercise discretion about the timing of the following one – next week or next month or later. Is my habit subconsciously bringing them back earlier than non-gifters?

Most varieties of chocolate can be dealt with speedily, based on another principle: the sooner you succumb to temptation, the faster that temptation disappears. This system works with boxed chocolates containing a finite number of conveniently accessible goodies – say, twenty. They can be dealt with in two days, if I behave like a trained seal and pop a reward into my mouth after every patient visit. If I overindulge, "sugar-highs" followed by "sugar-lows" may make me appear a little intoxicated at times. It is bad form to have a silly grin on your face while a patient is enumerating a litany of problems.

When faced with a particularly annoying patient, I need a boost before the visit as well, and sometimes during the visit. The last is tricky, because it is impolite to chew in front of another person. The delicacy must be nestled in the mouth to melt slowly, only to be chewed softly when I am behind the patient's back during a chest examination. This process can take a particularly long time if Mrs. Caramel has been in, rendering me incapable of speech until the sticky stuff is removed from my teeth with the surreptitious help of a finger.

Physicians know that it's politically incorrect to describe patients by their disease – for example, "The hernia in room 441." Yet I have begun to label my special patients differently, including Mrs. Maraschino Cherries and Madame Truffles. Mrs. Hungarian Liqueurs covers all the bases. Her chocolate/alcohol combination can make me reel and stagger if taken all at once. With minimum effort I was able to convert Mrs. Dozen Bagels into Mrs. Two Snickers by telling her my home freezer was full of bagels. And after years of receiving alcohol from certain patients, I was able to convert them by telling them my own doctor forbade drinking.

My home life has suffered, of course. My wife is a great cook, and she finds it infuriating when making muffins to discover that her chocolate chips have disappeared. I even found her stash of semi-sweetened Baker's chocolate – not great, but not too bad in a pinch. The best find used to be chocolate icing, but once she caught me drooling, she determined never to buy it again. So much for licking the spoon. She also knows when I've been naughty outside the house, because of the sentinel pimple that tells her I've been into chocolate within the last forty-eight hours. That solitary zit on my cheek or chin leads directly to the doghouse.

My workday sometimes begins with hospital rounds, where I mooch chocolates in the nursing stations and at my patients' bedsides. After work I can reach for my stash in our downstairs fridge, on my way to the treadmill. At least I get some exercise while maintaining my chocolate blood-level. Unfortunately, the calories of energy being walked off are simultaneously replaced.

By now I have received four annual John Hershey bars. The first two were taken home, carved up, and donated to several friends at New Year's parties. The third was consumed by my wife and me, but the last one never made it home. I consumed it alone in a two-month Herculean effort just in time for Valentine's Day. Immediately replacements arrived from grateful yet unknowing and manipulated patients.

Update: John, also my patient, kept the Hershey bars coming for several more years, even after his mother died. They ended only when John himself passed away.

Snoozing sickness

It is a fact of life at medical conferences that many of our colleagues are asleep, especially after lunch and when the lights go down. To prevent this embarrassing lapse from happening to me, I once sat in the front row during a colleague's much-anticipated lecture. All I remember is her opening remarks and the applause announcing that the talk was over. The subject was the treatment of insomnia.

In our profession, we physicians sometimes hear grim details of a colleague's decent into decrepitude – as told to us both by our patients and by their children. I'll recount a couple of these sad stories – first the words of a concerned daughter about the last afternoon office visit she will ever make with her mother to the cardiologist Dr. X.

"As you know," she began, "Dr. X has looked after my eighty-five-year-old mother for decades, yet he barely seemed to know her as we walked in and sat down. His receptionist Amy needed to help him into his own chair, then stayed in the room to assist, as if her job depended on keeping him focused and conscious. It probably did. Unfortunately, the doctor had the wrong chart as he began his inquiries, leading to intense confusion as he reviewed tests that my mother had never had done and medications she was not taking.

"Amy caught the mistake and presented him with my mother's real file, the perusal of which caused intense yawning – not stifled yawns but full-blown mouth-wide-open noisy eruptions punctuated by repetitive questions. He asked Mom about her medications more than five times and seemed to find her answers quite humorous, his mouth forming a silly grin. Then he fell asleep.

"His eyes had narrowed to slits for thirty seconds before they closed completely. Mom and I politely waited quietly, listening to his gentle snoring. Amy was obviously embarrassed at his slumber and tried to jostle him awake, but to no effect. So she gave him a surreptitious pinch on the arm. Dr. X woke with an 'Ouch.'

"He shook his head and slapped his cheek a few times in a desperate effort to recover consciousness. When he finally spoke, he tried to regain his dignity and remedy the situation. Unfortunately, his comments were disjointed and totally unrelated to any previous conversation. It seemed as though he was describing a brief dream we had interrupted.

"Dr. X dismissed us and told us that my mother's family doctor would receive his conclusions and recommendations. This consultation had taken ten minutes, during which he was incommunicado half the time. He yelled at Amy to bring the next patient in as we escaped without bothering to make a follow-up appointment."

When my patient and her daughter visited me, I went over Dr. X's consultation report with them. It looked official but bore little relationship to what had actually taken place. Perhaps Amy wrote it.

Another patient, a depressed young woman, recounted how her psychiatrist had fallen asleep during most of her visits, leaving her to worry about his health and safety. She finally found the courage to confront him with his behaviour. Patients will put up with a lot, but they do have limits. He apologized profusely, likely worried about an official complaint to his licensing authority.

I relate these cautionary tales hoping that Dr. X was just having a bad day and that the psychiatrist has spoken to colleagues or searched his literature for advice on maintaining consciousness for fifty-minute stretches.

I too have been to a physician who fell asleep on me, so deeply that he almost fell out of his chair. Because I suffer from occasional post-prandial drowsiness, I offer some suggestions that have helped me stay awake.

- It is easier to stay alert before lunch, so I book most patients in the morning.
- Eat a small lunch. Apparently carbohydrates are bad right now, while proteins are good, but a dietician might settle this controversy.
- Chocolate seems to have a soporific effect and must be avoided – a problem because chocolates remain a favourite gift for patients to bring to their physicians. Cherry chocolates with a liqueur filling are twice as deadly. Fortunately, only one patient gives me these delicacies – and I haven't the heart to stop her.
- Go for a walk after lunch to clear your head and start afresh. If pressed for time, just walk twice around your office building.
- Post-prandial drowsiness seems to abate by three in the afternoon. Book more patients after that hour.
- Eat a snack around 3 p.m. to get over hunger pangs and reboot your energy. I recommend an apple, which takes time and concentration to chew.
- Apologize to patients if they have watched you stifle a yawn unsuccessfully, especially if they begin to ask discrete questions about your sleep habits. Blame the yawn on a late night.
- Have a siesta, as millions of people in other cultures do. A nap is possible in a medical office only with the cooperation of staff. In our culture it is known as a power-nap – and twenty minutes of downtime goes a long way.

Snoozing physicians

A few years ago this blog drew many responses in the *Globe and Mail* "Patient navigator" section, which dealt with patients' questions about the doctor-patient relationship.

Medical doctors, psychologists, and various other psychotherapists often deal with angry and depressed clients. Many of these patients have conflicted and negative feelings about therapy to start with, so bad things can happen if the therapist falls asleep.

The column's writer, Lisa Priest, posed the question, and it drew some scary replies. Here is one of them:

"On several occasions my doctor has fallen asleep during our session. I see him nodding off, watch his eyes narrow to slits, see his head hang back and his mouth flop open, and, finally, hear him snore for up to a minute. There is no doubt that he is asleep. When he snaps back into consciousness, he looks bewildered and starts to spout gibberish about topics unrelated to anything we have been discussing. After a few minutes of sensible dialogue, I leave.

"My questions to you, Lisa, are: Is he getting paid for napping on the job? Do I shake him to wake him? Or do I call his secretary in? You may wonder why I keep going back. First, he helps me a lot when he is conscious, and second, by now I find this behaviour somewhat entertaining and exciting. He is getting pretty close to falling out of his chair, at which point I would prevent this from happening, though I am a rather frail woman.

"I wonder if I should report him to some authority. Is it ethical for me to take a video with my phone? I am sure that it would go 'viral,' but I really don't want to tarnish his reputation. I know that I should tell him about this falling asleep at every visit, but I am too embarrassed to confront him. Please help."

These are some of the more interesting comments sent in by bloggers, many of whom can be aggressive under the cloak of anonymity. The most obscene or vulgar comments were edited out by the newspaper. While most patients seem to be intimidated by this situation, others regard a sleeping physician as an opportunity for mayhem or theft.

Aggressive patients
- My therapist slept too, until I made a loud noise by clapping my hands. It worked, but when I explained my annoyance, he suggested that I would need a few more sessions about my anger issues.
- Once he is alert, he will be "all ears" when faced with something that is "very difficult to tell." He will think you are about to tell something juicy about yourself. Tell him that he fell asleep and that he does it frequently, and that you are very angry about paying him to nap. Suggest that he needs help. He will likely apologize and agree that this is a problem, or …
- He may become assertive and resume his healer role, asking, "How does my falling asleep make you feel?" You will respond, "Well, hurt, underappreciated, not respected, as if I am not worth your time." He may then say, "Let's explore the origins of those feelings." Now he is on familiar territory. No doubt he will try harder next visit.
- I don't want to be rude, but no wonder you are in therapy. Get a backbone and a new therapist. This is a problem only if you let it be one.

Intimidated patients
- Many clients of therapists are not of an assertive nature, and are easily intimidated like myself. My psychiatrist slept during my first twenty sessions, until I got the courage to mention this. He has been livelier since.

- If he takes offence at being confronted, you are in a very vulnerable position. He has the ability to discredit you by adding something to your personal file which is a lie. If you apply for insurance later, with your permission such information is sent to insurance companies and may be damning.
- Be careful what you complain about and how you do it. You should note that doctors compare notes and reserve special treatment for difficult patients. I learned this from watching *Seinfeld* on television.
- Although it is tempting to throw something soft at his head, you must remember who has the power here. If the therapist is a psychiatrist or other physician, he can have you locked up in a mental institution for aggressive behaviour.
- Leaving quietly would shift the onus nicely. If the sleeping is a ruse to demonstrate to you that you are boring, you will quickly find out. If not, you will get a call and an apology.

Practical patients
- The next time you have a session, you should sit in his chair and tell him to take the couch, where he will be more comfortable while asleep.
- Ask him if it would be OK to shake him or spray water in his face if he nods off.
- Slip some Ritalin into his coffee or offer him a high-energy drink such as Red Bull at the start of each session.
- By far the easiest way to deal with this is to print this column and show it to him.
- It is obvious that you should mention this serious concern. The sensible therapist will be apologetic and perhaps give an explanation about why this happens. Perhaps he is already seeing his own therapist. He certainly must see his own physician to rule out narcolepsy or sleep apnea.

Larcenous patients

- After he has fallen asleep at several visits, you could time the average nap and, with this information, admire the valuable keepsakes most physicians have in their offices and help yourself. Since he likely falls asleep with other patients, he will be unable to determine the culprit. Consider these objects barter for the valuable time he wastes while asleep with you. If he is seeing you for depression, your mood will improve with the prospects of future "presents."

Doctors who yell

Yelling at impossible patients is not recommended. I heard one doctor do so during my training, and it created great discomfort for everyone else in that outpatient department. Sadly, I have also witnessed a colleague who regularly lost his temper on hospital rounds and lashed out at patients, nurses, and other doctors. It was not a pretty sight. Cooler heads must prevail in our stressful profession, given the awesome responsibilities we all share. Fatigue and overwork are no excuse for incompetence or for rudeness.

I admit that, as a young and sensitive medic, I did raise my voice in anger, but these few incidents invariably led to regret and ruined the rest of my day. It also reduced my usefulness to those blameless other patients yet to be seen. Young physicians do not like to be second-guessed by patients or their families, whereas experienced physicians learn to calmly negotiate their way around disputes.

We serene and dignified older docs handle troublesome individuals by smiling and nodding politely while saying softly to ourselves, "This guy is a first-class idiot" or "This woman hasn't got a morsel of brain in her head." We just listen to the nonsense, then make rational and sensible comments leading to a prompt exit from the danger zone. Well – that is the theory.

Enter Mrs. Rose, at the worst moment of any family physician's day: high noon. By that time I'm hypoglycaemic, thirsty, and irritable, and exhausted from seeing too many additional "urgent" cases. By noon my head is swimming from making innumerable decisions and arrangements, and my arm is limp from writing prescriptions.

I'm sure I'm not alone in this midday morass. Most physicians know this condition well. Oddly enough, it can be cured in five minutes by an apple, eaten before the last hurdles of the morning must be leaped over. But too often I tend to carry on regardless of discomfort, trying to reduce waiting time for those last few patients.

It was during this moment of weakness that I lost it with Mrs. Rose. Not too loud, mind you, but I did raise my voice a little after she began giving me hand signals from the waiting room to speed up her visit and then declared, "I got to get back to my apartment – the cleaning lady's coming. Hurry it up."

With a tight smile I snapped, "I am delayed because I have been attending to patients who need more time, as you do sometimes. Emergencies happen. I think you can tell I have not been off on a long coffee break." Now, Mrs. Rose is a really sweet eighty-year-old who always bakes treats for us doctors and our staff before each visit. For some dumb reason I ended my tirade with these cruel words: "And you can keep your darn cookies. And your apple strudel too!" She was offended and told me so, but the office visit was concluded without more sparks.

When I phoned Mrs. Rose later that day to apologize, she accepted graciously but added: "You know doc, you were right. I was rushing you, and I won't do it again. The only thing I can't understand is about the cookies. What do the cookies have to do with anything between us?" That was a good question.

Mrs. Rose's next visit was anxiously awaited by all the office staff. Would she even show up? This question was answered by my secretary, who phoned her the day before the visit to confirm the appointment. Mrs. Rose was coming. Even more important, would she bake for us? Yes! She brought us a wonderful sampling of muffins and cupcakes, which we all thoroughly enjoyed.

Mrs. Rose's visit went well, and it ended with her on tiptoes reaching up to give me a big kiss on the cheek, signalling that all was forgiven. I wore her lipstick smear proudly the rest of the day: it seemed to throw all the ladies in the office into hysterics whenever we passed.

The next time a difficult patient deserves an education in medical etiquette, I will remember my incident with Mrs. Rose. At the very least, I will consider my opponent's culinary abilities before I shoot my mouth off again. My staff were ready to go out on strike if she quit my practice.

Hiccups

Hoping for a cure for hiccups before my next episode, I'm ready to confess to this embarrassing and debilitating problem. It's impossible to conceal from patients, and in a family practice where several patients are seen each hour, the possibilities for unintended buffoonery are obvious.

Usually caused by overeating or by swallowing fluids the wrong way, hiccups make it physically and mentally impossible to practise medicine properly. Because each spasm jerks the entire body from its intended course and leaves the brain briefly out of oxygen, it ensures that you not only look like a goof but probably talk like one too. Hiccups are likely to take the consultation in the wrong direction even as you also forget the patient's name.

I am not talking about a mild burp here. My hiccups are of industrial strength and are frequently associated with spilling coffee and dropping equipment. And anyone who wears spectacles can imagine how difficult it is to retrieve glasses from the floor without glasses on! I am left shaken and sweaty, slouched and moaning in my chair or leaning on a wall.

Talking makes things worse, but even a physician who is a good listener has to speak eventually. In my own case, my professionalism may wind up scattered all over my examining room, depending on where the hiccups took over.

Patients respond to my comical performances in variable ways. Some turn the doctor-patient relationship around by prescribing that I drink a glass of water, hold my breath, or apply cold spoons to my temples. If I am desperate by this time, I will let a patient supervise the cure. This reversal creates an odd and silent hiatus in a medical visit, filled with expectation and drama – and inevitably terminated by another round of discouraging hiccups I am unable to suppress.

One well-informed man told me to hold ice cubes or a cold soda can against the front and side of my neck, to deactivate my diaphragm's vagus nerve supply. As I had neither ice nor soda, this treatment must wait until next time. Another patient advised me to breathe into a paper bag in her presence, but I drew the line there and tried it out in private. Useless, again.

Patients who may have first heard my loud explosions from the waiting room are sympathetic only to a point. They are anxious to have a serious discussion with a real doctor, not some ninny who, after every sentence, makes a belch and says, "Sorry, I hope this will stop soon," or "Please excuse me, I'm really a mess – you know how hard it is to stop hiccups."

Answering phone calls in this condition is problematic too. This loss of control and resulting silliness offered to any colleague or other health worker gives the wrong impression. The caller may even imagine a very drunk or otherwise impaired physician. It's preferable to declare yourself temporarily out of service.

Surely I am not the only physician to suffer, but some may be able to hide this ailment from patients. In this group might be psychiatrists, if they work from behind a reclining patient, and hypnotherapists, whose entranced patients' eyes are closed. These doctors might be able to stifle their hiccups with difficulty. I doubt it, however, and can only imagine what their already sensitive patients must think.

I have never discussed this shameful dilemma with colleagues, but I am now convinced that hiccups are an occasional cause of patient morbidity and mortality. Imagine the surgeon whose scalpel slips while deep in someone's belly, or the gastroscopist who punctures the stomach lining and winds up looking at the spleen. Think of the damage that gynecologists or urologists might do with their probes in the wrong orifices, and the mayhem from a bronchoscopist who finds himself in the wrong lung. It is quite fortunate, all things considered, that I am not an eye surgeon or a heart surgeon.

The list is endless, and I suggest that fellow medical sufferers face up to this vile ailment and make this oath with me: "I will never face a patient while under the influence of hiccups. Though it may take an hour or more, I will bear the consequences of keeping patients waiting." We will not find support groups for this condition, so some discreet networking is definitely in order.

MIND GAMES

Beware of honest physicians – they may be dangerous

For a single day, Dr. Annie Davenport operated under a "truth serum" and spoke her mind freely to patients, without fear of hurt feelings or concerns about letters of complaint to her medical association. Normally, of course, she knew that the art and practice of medicine requires acting at many points through the day. Thespian-physicians have their "game faces" on as soon as they don their lab coats and their stethoscopes swing into action. However, while absolute honesty can be undesirable for anybody in certain social settings, it is a disaster in some aspects of the doctor-patient relationship. Any physician knows what I am talking about. We often suppress our true feelings, trying to be non-judgmental and kind.

And so the fun began: Dr. Davenport spent most of that day seemingly trying to destroy the excellent family practice she had nurtured for twenty-five years. Even her secretary, Linda, was ready to quit by noon, exhausted from consoling tearful patients as they left Annie's examining room. A satisfactory employee for ten years, Linda herself had come under severe and constant criticism that day. Medical secretaries occasionally feel the wrath of an employer's tongue when stress and frustration levels rise, but most physicians try to spare them. Secretaries also participate in the gallows humour needed to handle tougher cases. Not on this brutal day.

Annie's candour flowed from a mix-up in her prescribed medication. She had erroneously taken too much of drug A and too little of drug B. Her own family physician had given her these mood-altering medications. She arrived at her office late, looking angry and wild-eyed. She hustled through her packed waiting room and, without a hello to Linda, began tossing files around and mumbling to herself about all those patients who needed to be seen.

Her first victim was cheerful and unsuspecting Jane, a long-term smoker. Linda and the patients in the waiting room were alarmed to hear Annie yell, "Jane, look at yourself. At our age, fifty, you look ten years older than me. We have talked about your smoking for twenty years, with no effort on your part. Soon lung cancer or some other cancer will give you a prolonged and painful death." The examining room went quiet while the doctor caught her breath and then abruptly ended the visit, saying: "Don't bother to make a follow-up appointment. We have been playing games for about a hundred visits so far. I don't want to see you until you have stopped smoking, and since that will never happen, this is goodbye." Jane left the room in tears, without making an appointment, and departed with her head down. Had she looked up, she would have seen the mixture of fear and surprise on the faces of everyone else in the waiting room.

Into this gathering storm came Bill's wife, Brenda, the domineering half of a couple. Annie's patient was mild-mannered Bill, who had just retired at age fifty-five because of ill health. His scolding wife was not a patient, but she always invited herself into the examination room because, she claimed, "He doesn't pay attention and gets all your advice wrong." Other niceties were usually spat out loudly while glaring at Bill, who just shrugged and agreed with a silly grin from the safety of his perch on the examining table.

Brenda was also an "accuser," familiar to doctors as the sort who questions every bit of medical advice in this fashion: "Why didn't you treat him [her way] last week? He would be better already." Or "Don't give him that drug. You must know of its dangers. Don't you read the newspapers?"

On this day, Brenda was subdued because of the shouting she had heard. In fact, for once she stayed in the waiting room. Annie would have none of this modesty and beckoned sweetly with a crooked index finger for Brenda to join her husband. She started the visit with the caution: "Please remember that your husband is an intelligent adult and can manage without your constant criticism."

With a tight smile she went on, "And, since you continually question my advice, I would ask you to remember that I have treated your husband for twelve years, and he has done well so far. Please let me do my job." Finally, being on a roll, Annie remembered staff abuse, adding, "I would also appreciate if you would stop yelling at my secretary. Criticizing her for an inconvenient appointment time is cruel because she cannot fight back. Let her do her work too."

Spent from her efforts, Annie told Brenda to scram. As the chastened wife hurried out, she saw Linda standing up, punching the air with her fist, and exclaiming "Yes, yes!" The fallout from this scene actually worked: Brenda never screamed at Linda again, and Bill stood six inches taller on his later visits. On those rare occasions when Brenda did show up, she remained silent.

That is how the morning went, and it ended with Annie snapping at Linda about phone calls and repeat prescriptions to be dealt with. She gobbled lunch in the five minutes left before her first afternoon patient arrived, having lost an hour because of her tardiness and her agitated pacing about the office. Her "lectures" had been swift and surgically incisive, so the delay had certainly not been caused by her spending more time with patients.

That afternoon had a genital twist. Good-looking Peter, a forty-year-old accountant, had turned up with yet another venereal problem, but he felt confident about his chances for prompt relief. As he related his symptoms, Annie's rage was evident in both her demeanour and the loudness of her grunts. Peter became alarmed. "You make me sick!" yelled Annie. "You have a good wife and fine young children, and you screw around with other women. Peter, this is your fourth episode, and I won't cover for you this time. If your wife calls and asks me why I told you to avoid marital relations for a week, she will get the truth." As this message was delivered fortissimo, Peter cringed, thinking about facing the other patients. Annie ended the visit, saying, "Don't bother to take off your clothes – I don't want to touch you. Go to the VD clinic downtown."

"Next patient!" Annie called, peering into the huddled mass of fearful individuals in the waiting room. She repeated it twice, but no one had the guts to stand up. Linda then asked everyone to leave, saying their doctor was ill. They understood: some expressed concern, and they were all happy to get out of there. Linda then spoke quietly and tried to comfort Annie. In ten years, her employer had never before raised her voice. At first she was told to mind her own business, but soon Annie melted and released her frustrations as they sat together. She confided in Linda about her stresses with her partner, her parents, and her career.

Annie soon calmed down, first with a light touch and finally with a gentle hug. Linda had seen the doctor work this magic countless times with patients in the past. Patients with extreme anxiety and depression had often left the office with a smile and a livelier step, drying their tears. Wisely, Linda had cancelled the last few appointments of the day and had called Annie's own doctor, in the same building. She sat with her in his waiting room until he saw Annie and advised her at length. He insisted that she take the rest of the week off – unthinkable for a stressed physician – but she did.

The lesson? No matter how tempting it is to be completely honest and say exactly what you think, it can be demoralizing or even deadly for your patients.

Bizarre coincidences in medical practice

We physicians know that puzzling coincidences occur frequently in our professional lives. I have discussed this phenomenon with colleagues, so I know that I am not the only doctor who seems to be endowed with special powers. For example, certain patients will call for an appointment the day after I thought of them, usually after a long absence. Every physician has experienced this strange connection of thought processes between two persons. It is common among lay persons as well. However, far more bizarre things have been happening to me.

To begin, I must state categorically that before I met John I had never been an employee of Bell Telephone. John, aged forty, was referred to me several years ago by his then family physician. This doctor took the unusual step of phoning me before John's first visit – a hint, I suspected, that I was about to receive a real prize.

"John is schizophrenic," he began. "He has had several admissions to hospital, prompted by hallucinations and delusions, aggravated by non-compliance with his medication. He is currently stable and working because his concerned wife watches him take his antipsychotic drugs every morning and supervises his daily routines."

I listened carefully as the physician went on. "John's main delusion when he is ill is that Bell is running his life through all the phones in the house as well as light fixtures, air vents, radios, television, and other appliances. He feels that his physicians are part of this plot, but he usually goes along with their advice, despite his paranoia."

One minute into John's first office visit, I was interrupted by a personal phone call from a friend who works at Bell, calling to arrange a golf match at a Bell-sponsored event. I maintained my composure with some difficulty as we spoke. Luckily, I was not on speakerphone with my friend. If John had heard this exchange, he would likely have fled, and I would not have blamed him.

In the last few years, John and his wife have lived up to their description. He is a well groomed and intelligent man who appears normal in every respect, and he tries to reassure me on the subject of his mental illness, denying it all. His wife later tells me that he still occasionally talks to his light bulbs when he thinks that she is out of the room. For now, John takes his drugs, and his wife accepts his stability with relief.

And I await further instructions from Bell.

Deconstructing Michelangelo's *David*

A few months ago, as I looked at a picture of Michelangelo's *David*, I reflected on how much damage a malicious physician could do, using modern medical theory, to that magnificently sculpted body. Time was no object: he was already about five centuries old, and I still had a few pill-pushing years left in me. Long experience has taught me that I can mimic most illnesses by misusing drugs, then treat the iatrogenic problems with still more drugs. I rubbed my hands gleefully at this prospect.

David resides in Florence, Italy, and I live in Toronto, so it was obvious that my malign efforts were but wishful thinking. None of it applies in any way to my practice of medicine in the real world. My patients are safe with me, even though many of them are on some of the 250 commonly prescribed drugs I could choose from for my experiment.

To begin, I withered *David*'s muscular legs and arms by giving him a statin, a cholesterol-lowering drug, and telling him to take it only with grapefruit juice. From several options I chose the drug most known to cause rhabdomyolysis at high doses. Statins are now recommended by some authorities even for people with normal fat levels – for "pre-hyperlipidemia" – to prevent vascular disease.

Before long *David* would begin to complain of aches in his body and his limbs – a warning of muscle damage that of course I ignored.

A non-steroidal anti-inflammatory drug (NSAID) and a steroid itself fixed his muscle pain. I chose one of the first available NSAIDs, widely known to cause bleeding ulcers, and denied him the gastro-protection of a peptic acid inhibitor. Soon he was in so much abdominal pain he was doubled over, more than halving his fifteen-foot-tall frame. We now saw eye to eye. I quickly ignored his complaint of passing dark stools, often the first sign of internal bleeding from an ulcer.

When Vioxx was removed from the market in 2004, patients in Canada were encouraged to bring their supply back to their pharmacies for disposal. However, when the drug representative arrived to take my remaining supply, I lied and told him I had none, conveniently ignoring a full case unloaded by a different representative months before.

Had I given *David* my now contraband Vioxx, his decline might have taken longer. Still, after months of hiding his steadily increasing blood pressure, I had prepared the way for him to have a stroke or an acute myocardial infarction.

In the fullness of time, the ulcer caused fatiguing anemia, unknown to me because I neglected to test his blood or his stool. When he stepped off his pedestal to come to my clinic, *David* found his life energy much depleted, and his hands dragged on the ground, ape-like, to my hidden satisfaction.

The NSAID also raised his blood pressure. Some authorities have coined the phrase "pre-hypertension," meaning those cases where the systolic BP is 130 to 140, so I could get away with anything here. *David*'s BP responded nicely to a calcium channel blocker, but that swelled his shapely ankles. This problem I treated with a diuretic, knowing it was useless, and before long he was limping along with a rip-roaring hot foot from gout. Instead of stopping the diuretic, I added a beta-blocker to further sap his energy and libido.

David's chest interested me next. For his "pre-angina," I prescribed an ACE inhibitor, by now widely touted to give hypertensive patients the edge in heart disease, well before they have any symptoms. It led to a violent cough harsh enough to threaten his marble torso. The steroids further weakened his bones by causing osteoporosis. I could now crush his massive cold right hand with a strong handshake.

Turning my attention next to *David*'s pitiable psyche, I noted that he was justifiably depressed and that he had stopped sleeping. I therefore gave him a hefty daily dose of benzodiazepines, which deepened his depression. When that stopped working, I doubled and then tripled his dose, which strengthened my hand for the next course of treatment. I gave the poor man a modern antidepressant, carefully selecting one that led to agitation and an increase in his insomnia.

I was no longer envious of *David*'s universal sex appeal because the antidepressant removed his libido and the beta-blocker had caused erectile dysfunction. This once lusty man was too sick to notice any woman in my waiting room. Because the steroids had shrunk his genitalia, his fig leaf was not needed for anyone's modesty.

I could have justified giving him male hormone replacement therapy at this point. He now had symptoms that are supposed to drive us to prescribe testosterone: fatigue, soft bones, sexual difficulty, among other vague and common complaints. My contraband supply of estrogen HRT was unnecessary for *David*. He had been nicely neutered without it. He was far beyond asking for Viagra or its cousins.

His only chance of recovery now lay in non-compliance with my orders, but this idea never crossed his befuddled mind, given my sparkling reputation as a healer. He was instead grateful for all the attention he was receiving from me – about once a week for close observation. He had also received money-saving unlabelled samples from my overflowing drug cupboard. My ingenious nine-drug cocktail of statins, steroids, NSAIDs, antihypertensives, depressants, and antidepressants remained circulating in his diminished bloodstream.

By this time I was done. In a few short months I had succeeded in turning Michelangelo's *David*, the ideal of youthful manliness, into a hunched-over and hacking, pain-ridden zombie who could not even put his shoes on. And I was blameless. I had done most of my damage by following current recommendations, treating diseases he did not yet have and might never have. My failure to recognize adverse drug reactions made me just one of countless physicians who make a living in this way.

Flesh-and-blood patients had better beware.

DRUG REPS, DRUG COMPANIES, and PRESCRIPTION PADS

Drug reps bearing flattery, adulation, and praise

I have achieved every man's dream. Several times a month beautiful young women smile brightly at me as soon as they see me from the waiting room. Each asks anxiously if I can spare a few minutes for her. Should I agree, she picks up her mysterious attaché case and follows me into my consulting room, closing the door behind her. In this private setting she hangs on every word I utter, nodding in agreement. Flattery, adulation, praise, I get it all. Even if I say something dumb, common to many men in the presence of beauty, she lets it pass. She laughs heartily at my weak jokes and pretends to be in the presence of genius when I address scientific issues about drugs.

No, this well-dressed woman is not a medical groupie like the female fans attending on rock stars or baseball players. She is a highly educated pharmaceutical representative, and she humours me along until she can advertise her products and make them distinct from the competition. At this point the drug rep opens up her huge case, revealing it to be full of valuable samples. Out may come anti-inflammatory drugs, birth control pills, antidepressants, or sedatives. She may then extract a new antibiotic that neither she nor I can pronounce properly.

There are many pharmaceutical companies, most of which produce copycats of the more essential drugs. About half the reps offer me something for hypertension, for which there are now over fifty effective drugs. These drugs all work, so which do I prescribe? The reps are influential to some degree, as they leave samples for our patients. Most reps are promoting very similar drugs, give or take minor differences in chemical structure, so they have to make their products sound special and preferable.

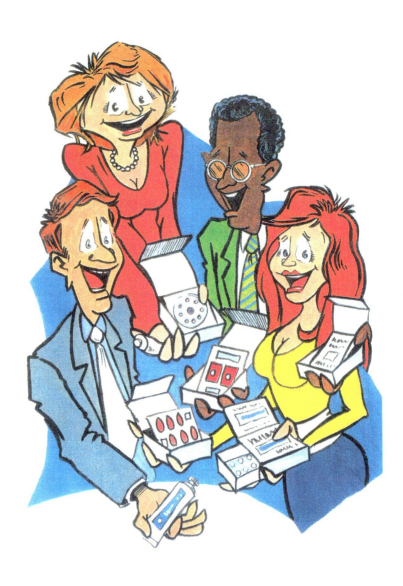

134   *Drug reps, drug companies, and prescription pads*

At this point the vivacious and enthusiastic rep passes scientific documentation across my desk and begins her sales pitch. Without doubt, some of it is said by rote, depending on how well she was trained. She extols her drug as the best, by virtue of half-life (the length of time it takes to degrade by half), lipid solubility, protein binding, fewer side effects, and so on. Like most physicians, I am weak on the basic science involved, so these facts sound good to me – at least until the next rep tells me something different.

All this attention can be very persuasive to a guy who had trouble getting dates in high school, but it ends after our ten minutes in seclusion, when the rep passes me her valuable samples after I sign her order form. She then leaves with a big smile and a firm handshake, happy with my tentative promise to consider prescribing her company's drugs. I tell each rep I will give her samples a try, but that is a fib: I stubbornly stick to one drug in each class until stronger evidence is sent my way.

Many of the current crop of male reps also seem to be exceptionally athletic and attractive – some even as Tom Cruise lookalikes. They would certainly qualify as "hunks" for a female audience. Though they work for different pharmaceutical companies, reps of both genders seem to be hired by personnel directors with a keen eye for beauty or masculinity. Is that a sales tactic by some drug companies? Have they spent a portion of their research budget concluding that a pretty face is an advantage with male physicians? And do they reserve the jocks for female doctors? My similarly impressed physician pals and I have discussed these issues at great length at meetings.

The reps and I get along well, and, if time permits, they are a welcome break in office routine. Because some are young enough to be my children, we chat about universities and their backgrounds. Their samples come in handy for uninsured patients, but their persuasion is also a great deal for the drug company they represent because I may be convinced to prescribe its drug for many future patients for years to come. Reps visit scores of physicians in their geographic areas, and no doubt every rep gets an occasional bad reception from a cranky or overworked doctor. Some promote excellent drugs that sell themselves, but others have to sample agents that are useless or even dangerous. It is no easy task to do so with skeptical physicians who are well aware of adverse drug reactions.

Sometimes a nervous new rep will appear with an instructor, who will supervise the visit with me. At these moments I am very kind and willing to sit patiently through tense detailing sessions even when the poor novice drops samples all over the floor. It is not surprising that reps from different companies may show up at the same time. Would it be too mischievous if I asked them to debate the relative merits of their products? Winner take all, as I promise to use her drugs forever.

How do the reps know if we really prescribe their products? Sadly, it has recently come to light that some drug companies have been purchasing computer printouts from pharmacists detailing each local physician's prescribing habits. This practice is controversial, and a battle is raging among the leaders of the drug triad: drug makers, drug vendors, and drug prescribers. Naturally, the Canadian Medical Association is opposed to this invasion of privacy.

Why are all these reps knocking on my door? Family physicians are the focus of attention for drug companies for two main reasons. We are the main prescribers by virtue of our numbers – currently close to half of all Canadian physicians – and we tend to treat the elderly, the group most in need of medication. The bottom line is that many newer drugs now cost $2 for each dose, and many of my older patients are on five of these drugs and several cheaper agents daily. Simple math shows an annual cost to Ontario's provincial health plan of $4,000 for that alphabet soup for each such patient. That spectacular reward is probably why these reps keep smiling at me. And here I thought it was my charm and good looks!

Drug companies bearing gifts

It is common knowledge that pharmaceutical companies have a large budget for the promotion of their products to physicians. They carry out this part of the business through their representatives and through sponsoring continuing medical education (CME) for physicians. There are firm guidelines about what favours drug companies can extend to physicians, but sometimes I wonder whether these ethical standards are followed. The more egregious freebies have now been eliminated. All journal articles must carry disclosures if the researchers are receiving payments from companies whose drugs are favourably mentioned.

Physicians often wonder if they have been affected by the promotional activities of pharmaceutical companies. I feel flattered by all the attention I receive and no doubt I am influenced, but not always in healthful ways for me or my patients. For example, I was recently invited to an industry-sponsored CME evening in a very fine restaurant – the kind I would not normally patronize. Going out at night after a busy day at the office was itself stressful.

I was greeted effusively by the pharmaceutical representative who had invited me. She had not only chosen the speakers and the venue but decided on the guest list as well – inviting any doctor with a pulse, it seemed. Over rich hors d'oeuvres and alcohol, I spoke to some physicians who said they attend many of these functions. Their lipid and energy levels must differ from mine.

Business began when the rep introduced a prominent cardiologist – and I hear he gave an excellent lecture. I had already eaten too much, however, and dozed off as soon as he showed his first slide. If I had fallen out of my chair, I might have been injured, but even that dreadful funk of drowsiness, accompanied by head nods and jerks, was frustrating enough.

When we adjourned for dinner, we were served delightful but breaded appetizers, followed by a thick steak with side dishes, and then ice cream with thickly iced cake. I ingested more fat that night than in a week of home-cooked meals. If I saw a patient indulging so, I would have yelled at him. Death by blood-vessel blockage threatened. I have read that such a meal can lead within hours to a boost in blood lipids and death. That evening got me thinking about my health. Here are my observations, based on that particular day in my life when I took advantage of all the industry activities and paraphernalia freely available to me.

At breakfast I chose reading material from one of the many medical journal obelisks scattered around my house. Some have reached the ceiling and are supporting the second floor. They have turned my domicile into a "local traffic only" zone. Fortunately, my wife and sons can negotiate from room to room without pushing a column over and sustaining crush injuries. Visitors to our house need to be guided through the clutter. No doubt many of my colleagues also get behind in their reading. Keeping up with the innumerable journals and drug-promotional articles we receive is a full-time job in itself. Most physicians are compulsive and perfectionist, so we don't throw literature out until it is properly processed. As a result, several inches arrive and are added to these columns every week.

Breakfast was stressful, as I chose a tabloid with surgical horrors on the front page. Indigestion followed as I persevered and read the entire article, along with some ads. Being of a suggestible nature, I always feel miserable seeing those severely depressed models in the antidepressant ads. While shaving I listened to a free audiotape. I cut myself badly trying to concentrate on some exotic facts that the speaker was discussing. The bleeding didn't stop easily because I have no time to shop for styptic pencils. While showering, I turned the tape's volume up and nearly electrocuted myself. In my car, I became confused and frustrated upon hearing conflicting glowing reports about two different lipid-lowering drugs on that same tape.

At my hospital, the first person I saw was a drug rep, and I chatted with her about her products. As usual I had trouble saying goodbye. In truth, I was taken by her beauty and had some dangerous thoughts, causing my pulse and blood pressure to jump. Fortunately, a colleague came by and allowed me to make a graceful exit. On rounds, to find my patients, I used my worn-out "red book" from one of the drug companies, outlawed several years ago by ethical guidelines.

The morning office ended late enough to make me rush through lunch. I read my mail while I ate and found two more wretchedly depressed models. By 3 p.m. I was more alert, but I soon had to contend with two drug reps from different companies talking about their nearly identical products. I was tempted to see them both at the same time, though that would have been cruel. Again I had trouble ending these rep detailing sessions.

After my office, much delayed, I hastened to the dinner CME meeting mentioned above, distracted by that same tape and annoyed at being late. Driving a bit too fast added to the possibility of an accident going to the meeting, as did two glasses of red wine for the road home. The discussions ended quite late at the hotel. Back home, energized by the food and drink and the collegial atmosphere, I slipped an industry video into my VCR. Later I fell asleep reading journal ads. Having been overfed and overly stimulated, even my sleep was affected. Predictably, I dreamed about juggling all those multicoloured tablets and capsules that constantly compete for my attention.

Fortunately, the next day was Saturday, a respite from my office life. Except for the journal obelisks.

Drug dreams

On very rare occasions, some doctors get attacked in their offices. One of my fellow interns was shot in an outpatient department when he told a patient she was pregnant. Disgruntled or psychotic patients have wielded knives – even a bow and arrow in one instance. A few abortion-performing doctors have been shot in their homes. Drug-crazed thieves are always a worry.

Still, all these misadventures could not explain my nightmare about a bizarre and frightening confrontation with a number of pharmaceutical representatives. Seated around the periphery in my own waiting room, occupying every chair, were about ten handsomely dressed young men and women. I knew them all: they were drug reps from a variety of competing drug companies, strangers to each other – or so I thought.

I had always made each of them comfortable during their drug detailing sessions, and until now I thought they respected me and my opinions. But this time no one was smiling, expect for me, and I was seated in the centre of the room with a tentative and quizzical half-grin at best.

In my dream, I next saw the reps taking drug samples out of their large briefcases and gently tossing them into an oversized green garbage bag, which I was holding open in the middle of the room. An alphabet stew of medications was about to teach me a new meaning of the term "drug delivery systems."

I watched as a cheerful, rather euphoric rep told me that she represented the manufacturers of the newer antidepressants. With a big, bright smile she tossed her stimulating mix of Luvox, Paxil, Prozac, and Zoloft into my sack. "No more sad days for you, doc," she chirped, before introducing a bilious sort who tossed in all the stomach remedies, from Losec to Nexium. He said a word or two about ulcers and heartburn, then belched loudly as he introduced the rep beside him.

Things took a decided turn for the worse when this woman began to fling round plastic birth control packages at me – Frisbee-style. She then used a slingshot to propel huge effervescent calcium tablets into my bag, just missing me in each case until one shattered on my forehead. The powder half-obscured my vision as it floated down to my glasses. Her specialty was women's health issues, but her quarterly visits to encourage me to prescribe more hormone replacement therapy had fallen on deaf ears. Her role in my dream ended ominously as she removed my lab coat, rolled up my sleeve, and stuck an estrogen patch on my bare arm, saying sternly, "Don't forget, the way to a woman's happiness is through hormones."

There was a pause in the action, and, as I looked around my waiting room, I caught my breath. I saw that a few reps were loading pea shooters, similar to the blow guns used by Amazonian Indians. Each of them in turn propelled several multicoloured oblong capsules at me at high speed. A few missed the bag, and I felt their sting on different parts of my body. From another direction, a kaleidoscopic collection whizzed by my head, close enough to comb my hair.

In a way I was being stoned, and I may have deserved it: I had not been entirely honest with some of these reps. I had accepted their samples and obligingly told each of them I would give the drugs a try. That was impossible, of course, but I could never say no to their persuasive arguments, especially if the detail came from a pretty face.

My custom is to stick with a single drug in each class, as long as it seems to be doing the job. This approach is safer for patients, as it means I am familiar with the drugs I prescribe. But it is frustrating to those who are promoting newer medications.

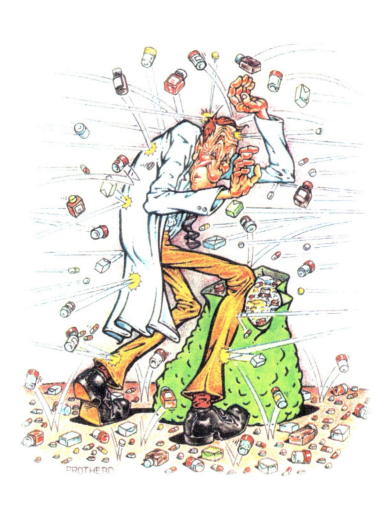

142 *Drug reps, drug companies, and prescription pads*

As if to prove this point, I watched as a hacking and oedematous foursome tossed in a mix of twenty-five excellent but roughly equal high-blood-pressure agents, from Adalat to Atenol to Zestril. They jostled each other and even me as they struggled to get my attention.

In the dream, as fresh troops marched in, each wearing a sneer, this first group began to leave my overcrowded waiting room and occupied the corridor. I knew these replacements well. One urgently added an ABC of urinary antibiotics, Amoxil and Bactrim and Cipro, then rushed off to my washroom. A lipid rep added her entire artery-opening collection, from Crestor to Zocor. One man began to smoke, then rolled up my other sleeve and stuck the various anti-smoking patches on my upper arm with his stained fingers. His hair and body smelled foul, and when he tried to talk, he could only hack and spit.

Beside him sat a fellow smoker who wheezed and struggled for breath as she threw several metallic and plastic inhalers at my bag. One ricocheted off my forehead as my perilous situation worsened. In an effort to calm me, my next assailant sleepily added the twenty or so available tranquilizers and hypnotics to my bag. "You look a little tense, doc," she said. "Try some of these pills. Are you getting enough sleep? Take them and you won't wake up for two days."

For a new twist on the proceedings, a very seedy and flatulent rep opened a dozen containers of psyllium and poured in their contents. He was followed by an "arthritis expert" who hobbled in with two canes. He needed my assistance to dump his countless anti-inflammatories into my bag before I helped him sit down.

By then only one man was left, and I felt my ordeal must be nearly over. To my chagrin, however, he pulled a box from his briefcase which I instantly recognized as the huge syringe of depot Zoladex. This trochar could be lethal. He prepared to fling it at me like a dart when a woman's voice rang out, "Stop!"

I knew her very well as Polypharmacy. She had always adored my lavish but obviously not good enough prescribing habits. It had been her job to encourage me to try as many different drugs as possible for each patient. She was a rep manager, and after a few minutes of whispered consultation with her colleagues, she sat down at my side. She apologized to me, saying things had gone too far. It was all meant in fun, she claimed. At that point I laughed nervously. Big joke!

She then told the reps what they already knew – that I was a respected physician whose therapeutic expertise was beyond reproach. But she had one request: "Would you be willing to give some of the more recent medications a try?" Fearing for my life, I nodded and answered quickly in the affirmative.

She then announced to everyone that all was well. In my dream the mob cheered and applauded loudly, some coming back from the corridor to shake my hand vigorously and give me their remaining ammunition. My bag now weighed several kilograms, but one tall man had no difficulty in sealing it and suspending it from the ceiling of my waiting room.

I was puzzled until he handed me a golf club and told me to smash the bag, as though it were a Mexican piñata full of candies. On the first whack the thing exploded and showered everyone with drugs. All the reps applauded and cheered loudly as a pill fight commenced and they pelted each other. Finally I had a chance to retaliate. Then they left, leaving Polypharmacy and me alone to tidy up.

As we worked I asked her, "What would have happened had I said no to your request?" With a smile, she took a bottle of juice out of her purse and grabbed a big handful of drugs. "You would have been asked to swallow these pills."

A daring method of drug selection for the harried family physician

I have decided to prescribe drugs only if their names begin with the letter *A* or the letter *Z*. It's a survival tactic after many years as a family physician struggling to keep current on drug therapy and not really as odd as it seems: many pharmaceutical companies name their products beginning with *A* or *Z*. This phenomenon is also well known in commerce, where these letters are popular among taxi companies, contractors, and other businesses.

Countless dollars are spent by the pharmaceutical industry in trying to convince us physicians to prescribe their products. Much more is spent on salaries for their drug reps, who call on us regularly. Patients can spot them easily in any doctor's waiting room. They are well dressed and bright young men and women toting heavy briefcases. They never take their overcoats off because their mission is simple: a brief raid into my already overstimulated cranium. I listen politely and get detailed on the virtues of the particular drug company's medications, and then I accept free samples to try out on my patients.

But every successful drug in a new class attracts numerous copycats. There are now more than twenty anti-inflammatory drugs in the lucrative arthritis market, and well over fifty drugs for hypertension. I can't make every drug rep happy. Physicians are overcome with choices, but long experience has taught me that there is little difference among the drugs in the same class. They have the same function and carry the same potential side effects.

And so I decided to have some fun and simplify my life without endangering my patients. Instead of memorizing the trade name, generic name, strength, and dosage of several drugs for each indication, I now prescribe drugs based on their fortuitous appearance in the alphabet. If they work and are safe, no amount of persuasion or arm-twisting can alter my course.

On the Monday I introduced my revolutionary system, my first three patients were hypertensive. No fewer than three ACE inhibitors sprang immediately to mind – Accupril, Altace, and Zestril. Later, depending on the circumstances, I prescribed other hypertensive patients with the diuretic Aldactone, the beta-blocker Atenol, or the calcium channel blocker Adalat. I was really on a roll by then, and my excitement grew with each patient.

By Monday afternoon I had exhausted the first four classes of drugs, but hypertensive patients were still arriving. High blood pressure is by far the most common disease family physicians treat. Luckily I began to seek help from the ARBs (angiotension II receptor blockers). There were six to choose among, but I alternated Atacand and Avapro.

I ran into some trouble when I was faced with infections: Amoxil and Ancef can go only so far, and some patients are allergic to penicillin. The letter Z sprang to mind again, so I began to prescribe Zithromax for respiratory infections. In came a patient that afternoon with herpes zoster on her chest wall: quick as a wink I gave her Zovirax tablets, costing its competition several hundred dollars.

My timing on this decision was impeccable. When one well-read patient with high lipids demanded a statin, I immediately wrote a prescription for Zocor.

Mental illness was easily handled with my system. By Tuesday I was giving my depressed patients the older tricyclics Anafranil and Aventyl, or the SSRI inhibitor Zoloft (one of many similar drugs spawned by Prozac). One of my psychotic patients showed up that day, but his psychiatrist, a woman who obviously shares my system, had him well controlled on Zyprexa.

Benzodiazepine drugs are widely used as sedatives and sleeping pills, ubiquitous since Librium and Valium pointed the way to our narcotized society. About twenty different pills are available, but my job was made easy with Ativan. For a patient who had not responded in the past, I gave Zopiclone, of a different class called "Z-drugs"!

An Alzheimer's patient came in Wednesday. After a lengthy visit with his children and wife, I confidently advised them that Aricept might slow down the progression of his disease.

By Thursday I had seen many patients with chronic pain and many with arthritis, but I handled them easily with Acetaminophen, Anaprox, and Arthrotec. Without a second thought I gave a stooped-over osteoporotic lady Actonel to strengthen her bones.

Anyone who burped that day was given the antacid Amphojel. If they were really suffering from their reflux and heartburn, I prescribed Axid or Zantac, both potent acid inhibitors.

Aspirin was already my favourite anticoagulant. Acarbose and Avandia were enlisted to solve my diabetics' problems. Amcinonide cream comforted all my eczema patients that week, and Alesse protected some of my young female patients from pregnancy. Everybody with sniffles got Allegra, everyone who itched got Atarax, and everyone who wheezed got Advair or Atrovent.

An alcoholic smoker was my last patient on Thursday. I was rather exhausted by then with my new game, so I impatiently gave him a double-whammy of Antabuse and Zyban, aiming to cure both his bad habits at the same time. I told him to stop immediately if this combo's listed side effects occurred. I certainly did not want him to stop breathing.

Friday came soon enough, and by then my head was swimming with *A*s and *Z*s. I was really having fun, and as luck would have it, rarer and miscellaneous categories of illness turned up. I gave a migraine-headache sufferer Zomig, a gouty patient Zyloprim, and my patient with prostate cancer got his regular injection of Zoladex. I took careful notice that dermatologists were still using Accutane for acne, and that one gastroenterologist was keen on Asacol for colitis.

The first week using my system was nearly over, but for a young man who threatened to alter my revolutionary system of drug selection. Resentfully I listened to his story of erectile dysfunction (ED) and his desire for Viagra, Cialis, or Levitra, none of which were acceptable to me that week. As we talked, I got a last-minute brainwave. Why not give him something for a condition called Low T, a new invention of the drug industry? Low testosterone was by then blamed for ED, soft bones, and weak minds. Ordinarily I would do things scientifically and test his testosterone level before prescribing, but it was lunchtime and I had to get ready for a big golf game. I easily talked him into the latest topical testosterone product, Axiron. Then I realized he was a smoker – very bad news.

I had to tell him of the dangers of Axiron. When applying and wearing this solution, he could not go near an open flame. I cautioned him not to light up a cigarette post-sex: if he exploded, the expected afterglow could become a disaster. Moreover, if his female partner were to come in contact with Axiron, she might grow a beard and break out with horrible acne. I advised him to use this drug only in his armpits, which no one seems to consider an erogenous zone.

And so the week passed, and I caught my breath that weekend. I had narrowed my list of available drugs down from well over two hundred to around fifty and greatly simplified the practice of medicine for me. The letters *A* and *Z*, I thank you.

Goldilocks revisited

Once upon a time there was an elderly white-haired lady named Goldie who lived in a small apartment. She was unhappy because her husband had died long before, and her only child, Joanie, did not visit her very often.

As Goldie grew more depressed, she lost her ability to sleep properly and never got enough rest. She went to talk to her doctor about her nervous problems, but he seemed to have an anxiety problem of his own. Rather than discuss what was bothering her, he gave her some "happy-pills" and some "sleepy-pills" and said goodbye after five minutes.

Like any good patient, Goldie took her pills, but after a few days something very scary happened. She woke one morning and smelled something cooking on her stove. After a look in her kitchen, she panicked and phoned the doctor to hurry over: she needed his help. Because this is a fairy tale, he made a house call.

After the doctor stepped off the elevator on her floor, he walked along the corridor, and his nose detected the delightful aroma of chicken soup. He followed its trail right to Goldie's doorway. "Oh good," he thought, "Goldie will give me some of her soup."

The doctor noticed that Goldie was still in her nightclothes and still quite distressed. She led him into her dining room, where he found her table beautifully set for six people, plates and silver shining. One bowl contained some soup and a spoon, and the napkin beside it had been used. Then Goldie took him into her kitchen, where he found the simmering chicken soup that was making her so sad.

Goldie began to cry, her great tears splashing into the soup. "Doctor, I did not set my dining-room table and I did not defrost this chicken. I think a burglar came into my apartment during the night, cooked the soup, and laid the table. The burglar then sampled the soup and left my apartment with the stove still on."

After Goldie had cried some more, she composed herself and continued with her story. "I have already phoned my daughter, Joanie, and I've got her worried. She hasn't been to visit me for a month, so she wasn't the one who did this cooking. She's coming right over."

Goldie next led the doctor to her bedroom, where he spotted the clue to this mystery – her nearly empty pill bottles. "Goldie, I think you took too many of your happy-pills and sleepy-pills. You probably forgot that you had already taken these medications, and then took them again and again."

As Goldie thought about this explanation, the doctor went on. "I think you were sleepwalking last night, sort of in a trance. You woke up and did the cooking and everything else, then you went back to sleep. When you woke up a few hours later, you had forgotten all about your busy night."

This explanation sounded plausible to Goldie, so she began to smile. Her tears had dried by the time Joanie knocked on her door and came in with her husband and two young children. They all hugged Goldie and cried from happiness that she was all right. Goldie introduced everyone to the doctor, who explained the story to them.

The older grandchild then made a wonderful and very logical suggestion: "Let's eat the soup!" Even though it was an odd choice for breakfast, the doctor joined the family, and the six of them sat at the table until they had slurped it all up. As always, everyone felt great after chicken soup.

The doctor stood up and excused himself, and the family thanked him for coming over so quickly and helping Goldie. To himself, however, he said, "Wow, I will never give her so many of those pills again. I should spend more time talking and less time drugging. I am very lucky that these folks are not angry with me, because I was at fault." He left the apartment with a smile, waving goodbye to Goldie, who was enjoying the attention she was getting from her family.

Reconstructing Mary

We physicians are a dangerous lot. We can inadvertently raise blood pressure, damage the kidneys, ulcerate the stomach, shorten the breath, and race the heart. We can block the bowels, dissolve the muscles, clot the blood, weaken the bones, and disfigure or strip the skin. As if that isn't enough, we can depress the mood and addle the mind.

My new patient Mary confirmed that the biggest health hazard many patients face may be the earnest person in the white lab coat feverishly writing out prescriptions.

As we know, the second doctor on the case is always the genius because he knows which treatments were tried and failed before. In this case a sixty-five-year-old patient who was literally a toxic-waste dump was reborn. Her age was significant: as an Ontario resident, she had recently become eligible to receive "free" prescriptions. That benefit is sometimes a mixed blessing.

At Mary's first visit to me, referred by her concerned husband, she appeared to be a pale, depressed, and desperate woman. They told me that she had always followed her doctors' instructions faithfully – perhaps that was her problem. She could not guess that these doctors were making her ill.

Her presenting problem was headaches. I was concerned because new headaches at that age can signal the presence of a brain tumour or can warn that a stroke is on the way. During a recent hospitalization, however, all the exploratory tests they administered had been negative. Her previous family physician and her neurologist had tried her on eight different headache drugs, without success. Mary sat crying in my examining room, her aching head pounding in her hands, as her husband dumped all her regular daily medications on my desk. The very thud of these bottles made her wince.

One of these medications proved to be the cause of her grief. It was a lipid-lowering "statin" drug prescribed to Mary by her former family physician. I stopped it, and she was headache-free three days later.

The huge blue Compendium of Pharmaceuticals and Specialties (CPS) is the doctors' 2,500-page small-print "bible." We are expected to be familiar with all its contents – an impossible task. But countless patients could be miraculously healed if we physicians would only look up the side effects of the drugs we at times so cavalierly prescribe. My CPS spends a lot of my office time on my lap, thanks to Mary and others.

Was Mary annoyed with her physicians? Not really. Although we have this deplorable ability to make patients quite ill with a drug, we usually become the heroes when we recognize the error of our ways and stop the same drug.

Problems arise if we do not recognize the reaction for what it is and add to our patients' grief by prescribing still more drugs to fight the side effect. This phenomenon has been coined "the prescription cascade" by some clever colleagues because it can go on growing forever.

Getting back to Mary, I should explain that her situation was not as simple as I have portrayed. When she developed her "statin" headaches, she was also on several drugs for other chronic illnesses. This medley confused the issue considerably. She was also seeing specialists for some of her problems, and they added their favourite potions to the toxic brew circulating in her bloodstream.

Her mother had died of a stroke at age sixty, so Mary was eager to take the blood-pressure drugs that could prevent that disaster. Unfortunately, several drugs are needed in combination to control most cases, making this field fertile for adverse drug reactions. Predictably for Mary, she reacted poorly to her cardiologist's efforts.

Beta-blockers caused extreme weakness, her ACE inhibitors led to a severe hacking cough, and calcium channel blockers swelled her legs to the knees. I told her to buy a home blood-pressure monitor, so she could check her pressure daily. With those results in hand, I gradually stopped or reduced all three of these drugs. A month later she was a new woman. Her BP diary showed that she still had mild hypertension, but it proved to be manageable.

Mary also had arthritis. In the past, arthritis always hurt, but it became life-threatening only after the introduction of anti-inflammatory drugs (NSAIDs), which often cause upper gastrointestinal hemorrhage through ulceration. Mary was pale because she was anemic. She had been bleeding internally after her rheumatologist gave her a daily NSAID, but she pinked up once I prescribed iron tablets and different drugs for her arthritis. NSAIDs also raise blood pressure, and her doctors should have taken that side effect into account before they gave them to her.

During a later visit, Mary was still depressed about life, but her physicians were partly responsible for that too. The central nervous system (CNS) is quite vulnerable to drugs. In particular, tranquilizing drugs such as Valium and Ativan may cause depression because they are CNS depressant, but virtually any sort of drug can be mood altering and may convert patients to polypharmacy zombies.

Mary complained of fatigue, weakness, irritability, insomnia, and anxiety – all due to her combination of drugs from several doctors. She got better when we gradually reduced them and eliminated the Ativan a psychiatrist had prescribed two years earlier. Her overall improvement worked better than any antidepressant, so I discontinued her Prozac. She didn't need it anymore.

After a few months, Mary learned how to protect herself. She now insists that her pharmacist give her a printout of all her medications. And so in a way she became my assistant – sometimes spotting side effects before I did.

I too have inadvertently created lots of illness with my other patients, but that CPS on my desk enables me to make amends. All the drugs that gave Mary so much difficulty are valuable and harmless for most people – if they are prescribed responsibly.

My polydoctor patient

Polygamy is the practice of having many wives or husbands at the same time. Polydoctoring describes the practice of my patient Edith and her platoon of physicians. She is not unique, just one of many who take advantage of the generosity of the Ontario Health Insurance Plan (OHIP). Multiple doctors inevitably lead to dangerous polypharmacy.

As I sat taking Edith's history at her first visit, it became obvious to me that several of her significant illnesses were being handled by committee. Listening patiently to her account, I was surprised that she looked so well. She could have been investigated and drugged to death long ago as each physician was tempted to add a favourite medication or two.

If you put three doctors in the same room, you may get three differing opinions on any particular health problem. Just ask three urologists about the treatment of prostate cancer to prove this point. Edith, age seventy-five, put herself repeatedly at risk in this manner. It is difficult enough to understand and follow the advice of a single physician, yet Edith had offered up her pituitary and pancreas and thyroid to three different endocrinologists, perhaps one gland for each. She had entrusted her complicated cardiovascular system to three cardiologists, each with a set of stress tests and scans and echocardiograms. All six had been quite handy with their prescription pads. I knew about this excess because Edith had dumped her pill bottles in a pile on my desk, with some overflowing onto my lap. She fit the prescriber's name to each medication as her story unfolded.

I kept silent, with difficulty, as Edith checked her notes and progressed further down her body, naming the urologist and gynecologist who were dividing care of her urinary system, and the gastroenterologist and colorectal surgeon who had divided their spheres of influence neatly at her appendix. I pictured her orifices being scoped four ways at once to reduce anaesthetic time. When she paused to catch her breath, I could no longer restrain myself and spoke my mind: "You're seeing far too many doctors and you are on far too many drugs." This message went unprocessed and she asked, "May I continue now?" Eventually, I counted twelve consultants whom she had seen within the previous year, a full Canadian football squad of docs. Unfortunately, because they were all quarterbacks, this team had scored few touchdowns in her favour while defensively they had lost ground, each yard lost being an adverse drug reaction.

Still not fully satisfied, she had presented herself to me for interpretation and to "break some ties." No doubt her previous family physician was somewhere breathing a sigh of relief at this news while I prepared for the worst. I determined to use my low-tech skills, chiefly cerebral. As time passed after that initial visit, my attempts to simplify her life by eliminating excess drugs and doctors often alarmed her and sent her flying off for still more advice. One frustrated consultant commented: "We physicians have created a monster" by our ministrations, a dragon with an insatiable demand for doctors and drugs.

Consultants must resist the easy solution of referring to each other, once the patient overreaches the boundary of their specialties. Wiser specialists send the individual back to the family physician, who usually knows quite a lot about the previous medical attention. Under the present system, Edith is free to visit me and several other family physicians every week, without penalty. Her need for second and third opinions will come to an abrupt end the first time she has to pay for an unnecessary consultation. OHIP was wise to target such behaviour a few years ago with a ruling that patients cannot see a specialist without a referral from their family physicians.

A cautionary tale about vultures, fish, snakes, and devils on drugs

I have always been an unapologetic fan of *The Simpsons* TV show. All viewers of this famous animated sitcom know that the fish living downstream from the local nuclear plant have three eyes.

The *Globe and Mail* recently ran a story about research on fish on oxazepam, a sedative-hypnotic benzodiazepine similar to Valium. These fish depend on blending in with their fellows to avoid predators while travelling in schools. Research showed that fish with more tranquilizers in their system became aloof, unfriendly, and more apt to take risks. As a result, they were isolated and quickly snapped up. Does this personality change sound familiar? In his futuristic novel *1984*, George Orwell predicted a society in which the population was pacified by a drug called Soma. Our version is Valium and its twenty or so cousins, among them Ativan and Mogadon – all potentially depressing if prescribed and taken for more than the recommended two weeks.

Some time ago a lake fish near a big city was found to have five antidepressants in its bloodstream. I surmise it was a happy fish but easy to catch. Like over-drugged humans, it may have been swimming in circles or otherwise drawing unwanted attention to itself. We were not told which five antidepressants the fish was drinking, but my prescribing habits would suggest that Celexa, Paxil, Prozac, and Zoloft were in the mix. A significant percentage of North Americans are on antidepressants, and, because we all drink the same water as lake fish do, this story puts to rest the ridiculous proposition that antidepressants should be added to our drinking water along with fluoride. Guess what? They are already in our water.

Carp were dying in the thousands and washing up on the shoreline of Lake Simcoe cottage country in the summer of 2008. They are big fish, and homeowners often had bags of them at the roadside. They stank and represented another example of how any living creature could easily be wiped out. The theory was that carp and other species were poisoned after someone discarded a goldfish down the toilet or threw it in the lake. The toxic product this pet fish brought with it was a bacterium named *columnaris* – which is harmless to humans, at least so far.

Members of the ancient Zoroastrian faith in India rely on vultures to dispose of their dead, and the number of vultures has dropped precipitously. It turns out that some dead persons the birds had been eating were on anti-inflammatories. The birds cannot metabolize this drug, so they die. This class of drugs includes Advil, Aleve, Celebrex, and ibuprofen.

The Pacific Island of Guam has invasive brown tree snakes, introduced as stowaways on American battleships during the Second World War. The snakes have decimated bird life by eating their eggs. Wildlife officials in planes "bomb" the area with dead mice containing acetaminophen, which is toxic to snakes "and not a lot of other animals." The trade name of this drug is the ubiquitous Tylenol.

Finally, on the isolated island of Tasmania, just south of Australia, those fierce little Tasmanian Devils are now very prone to horrendous massive facial cancers, cause unknown, but they did not have this disease in the past.

As a family physician, I believe that we are exposed to any number of poisons when we breathe, drink, and eat. In Toronto, where I live and practise, some patients in their forties and fifties have had unusual cancers of the pancreas, stomach, bladder, breast, and large and small bowel – carcinoid tumours. Everyone I know seems to have family or friends in this age group who have developed cancer. The man who installed some cabinets for me came back six months later and forty pounds lighter – he'd had esophageal cancer.

We have a big problem here. We have known for decades that estrogen gets into our water supply from birth control and hormone replacement pills and that many toxic chemicals are converted to estrogen. Breast and prostate cancers are certainly hormone-dependent and show up in my mostly male practice as an abundance of prostate cancer in men in their sixties.

My patient roster includes hundreds of patients over the age of seventy-five, and oddly enough my older patients are doing well in terms of cancer. They still get it but in a less aggressive form than in younger patients. I believe that these elderly people, although they may have been deprived in many ways, were not exposed as children and teenagers to the environmental toxins that postwar baby boomers have faced.

There we have it. Things cannot improve unless we pay attention to the environmentalists, but they can get worse. Some high-risk women are having prophylactic mastectomies. Will there be a nightmarish future in which cancers are so common that our colleagues might advise young adults to remove their ovaries, uteri, testes, prostates, thyroids, colons, and gallbladders? No one wants cancer.

MEETING PATIENTS OUTSIDE the OFFICE

House calls – how to handle dogs, doors, and defunct doorbells

When I began my practice, house calls were very common. Few families owned two cars, and not many mothers worked outside the house, so they were home-bound. I had more children as patients then, and they were often seen at home. A house-call service covered physicians' practices after hours and on weekends, and I earned some extra income from this service in my early years as a doctor.

My adventures included driving into a ditch, running over a child's bike lying in a driveway, and having a child run and hide when I knocked on the door. The mother offered me a coffee while she tried to flush him out, but she was unsuccessful. I surmise he came out after I left. By that time the mother had figured out that if he was well enough to play such games, he didn't need my services. In high-rise apartments, there is always the possibility of elevator breakdowns. No one expects a physician to climb nineteen flights of stairs, but more than once I've had to navigate dark stairwells to exit a building.

Any doctor who has experience with house calls can relate some memorable moments. Here are some of the stories on my list.

THE WRONG DOOR: One of my first visits in an apartment building went very well. Looking as professional as I could at the age of twenty-eight, I completed the examination of my patient, gave my sage advice, and said my goodbyes to the grateful family. Then, as I tried to leave, I walked out onto the apartment's balcony! A snowy blast of cold air let me know that I had exited through the wrong door, as did the giggles of the children. Mustering my dignity, I followed them back through the apartment and out into the corridor. While waiting for the elevator, I heard them howling with laughter at my expense. Lesson learned: Always keep your exit plan in mind. You could just as easily walk into a closet or the washroom.

ANIMALS: The huge golden retriever accompanied me as I walked in through the unlocked front door and followed me upstairs to the patient's room. This creature had an obsession with my pelvic area, goosing me up the stairs, then sniffing around my privates as I conducted my examination. Finally I implored my patient to call his dog off, only to hear him say, "It's not my dog. I thought it was yours." Dog and I both left sheepishly. Lesson learned: Just because a dog is on someone's front lawn, never assume he's the family dog. That goes for cats as well, eager as they are for warm lodgings.

GETTING INSIDE: After a five-minute wait on someone's porch ringing a dead doorbell and knocking like a frustrated woodpecker, I finally had a great idea. I phoned my patient and said, "I'm on your porch. Please let me in – I'm very cold." Before cell phones, I was once reduced to tapping on a sleeping patient's bedroom window with a hockey stick I found in his backyard.

Lessons in patient avoidance

We all have a few patients who are very difficult to deal with, but we accept their peculiarities as a part of our job. We do not, however, have to give them a big "hello" should we see them outside the office. To illustrate my dilemma, I must explain that my office is near a shopping plaza in which I enjoy a lunchtime stroll. This habit puts me at the mercy of any annoying patients I might encounter, without the protection of my secretary and the security of my closed doors. Caught in the open, I would be easy prey were it not for my early military training.

When I was fifteen years old, my parents encouraged me to spend a summer at Camp Ipperwash with some school chums – to make a man out of me and to improve my posture. Neither happened, but as an army cadet I did learn various "survival" skills that have been valuable in patient avoidance. These stratagems would not work without the cooperation of the local merchants whom I have deputized.

My usual mission is to reach the bakery by 1 p.m., purchase my afternoon snack, and return to base by 1:30 for my afternoon patients. The easiest part is in the bakeshop itself, where most customers are busily engaged. If I see someone dangerous, Nina or Katerina behind the counter will fill my order based on hand signals. They understand that Mr. or Mrs. Patient might recognize my voice.

The real threat arises outside, in the plaza and parking lot itself, where patients spend a lot of time on a fine day, often with another patient or a spouse for double trouble. Some are making visits to the drugstore armed with the prescriptions I gave them that very morning.

One useful military manoeuvre here is the snappy "about-face," used to halt and turn oneself completely around while marching with one's platoon on the parade ground. This move must be done at the right moment, which is the instant the patient is identified. Any later, and the patient could be offended, having guessed the reason for this turn of events. It helps to rub the chin and furrow the brow during this routine, to give the appearance of having forgotten something important.

The turn-about need be done only if there are no easier alternatives. If I see an insufferable patient coming my way, I may cross the road to the opposite side, dart between moving vehicles, or pick up my pace to military "double time." Even these ruses can fail because many of my patients follow my advice to keep fit, and they can move pretty fast in pursuit of my free medical opinion.

Any soldier knows that knowledge of the terrain is essential. Shopkeepers help me out here, depending on where I am identified. Tony the barber knows enough to put me in a chair immediately if I signal that I have been spotted, and he will send me to the rear for a shampoo if he is too busy. Igor the shoemaker will hide me among his polishing machines, and Tom the Dairy Queen man lets me look busy with his hot-dog apparatus.

My biggest obstacle is the supermarket, where my superior officer (my wife) sends me on occasional missions behind enemy lines for some shopping. A few of my patients are almost always there, and the aisles are not long enough to do a successful about-face. Dodging from one aisle to another while crouched down and armed with a zucchini can look unseemly to checkout girls who know nothing about the infantry.

Things often go wrong in the military, leading to the inevitable snafu – a term that stands (approximately) for "situation normal: all fouled up." If well and truly captured, I mimic the "hands-up" position of a POW by a shrug and accept my fate. I do not, however, have to give more than my name, rank, and OHIP number. Medical information can be denied.

The beach, the mall, and the wedding hall

Patients can be very surprised to find their doctor out of his usual element. I know I was when, as a teenager, I saw my GP in an Eaton's department store with his wife and kids. "What's he doing here and who are those people with him?" I thought. After passing the time of day, I walked away astonished that my physician shopped, had married, and was raising a family. I could not conceive of him ever out of his office or the hospital, or without his white lab coat. Although many physicians are workaholics, we all have a life outside our medical spheres, and odd things happen when we meet patients in these settings.

I have never even considered what my physicians look like in swimwear, for instance, so I should not be surprised at my patients' reactions to me. Nora and Harry, an elderly couple, appeared to be shocked when I walked up to them on a Florida beach on the Atlantic Ocean. They were in up to their knees, wading and splashing quietly in the surf, when I appeared as a stranger clad in a swimsuit and a towel, with dark sunglasses and a big hat.

They were alarmed to see me approaching and wishing to shake hands but were relieved when I identified myself. We had a good laugh together. Doctors have every advantage in this situation because we are used to seeing our patients nearly bare. I recognized Harry's nasty surgical belly scar and his huge ventral hernia about a hundred yards before I saw his face. And not many patients have Nora's peculiar fat-distribution "thunder thighs." Amazingly enough, this combination of bodies would likely be found nowhere else in the world, and I was proved correct. They both seemed astonished that their family physician would have legs and arms like anyone else and that he could swim.

Coincidence reigns in medicine. For two weeks every winter for years I have been a beach bum on this stretch of sand and had never before seen any of my snowbird patients. Yet that same day, no more than two hundred yards further down the strip, I saw another elderly couple. I was smarter this time, not wishing to frighten them, so I loitered around a bit before saying hello. Anne and Morris were head down, looking for interesting shells. In view of my previous experience, I debated walking on by, but I did say hello, and we chatted pleasantly for a while in the sun.

None of these four patients asked me any medical questions. Perhaps the presence of the ocean and the novelty of our meeting spared me. I was trapped later that same week when I stumbled on a patient on the dry land of a shopping plaza. Bill was not too shy to tell me all about his kidney-stone attack, halfway into his several-week stay in Florida.

Ominously for me, just as I prepared to leave, we were joined by his wife, his brother, and his sister-in-law. They were all my patients, also halfway through a lengthy Florida vacation. At this point my patients often have a decision to make: Should they see an American doctor, who will charge them big bucks, or should they save their health problems for Dr. Rapoport back home?

Their prayers seemed to be answered when I materialized right before their shocked eyes. Thirty minutes later I had answered all their health questions while vowing to myself never to return to that particular mall. Relieved to say goodbye, I foolishly gave Bill my Florida phone number when he surprised me by asking for it. He didn't call, but I thought he might, and that is nearly as bad while on holiday.

My most embarrassing encounter with patients occurred during the wedding of a young couple in a residence for slightly disabled seniors, where a number of my patients had moved. To be honest, all of them had become difficult to treat in an office setting, and I encouraged them to attend the medical clinic in their

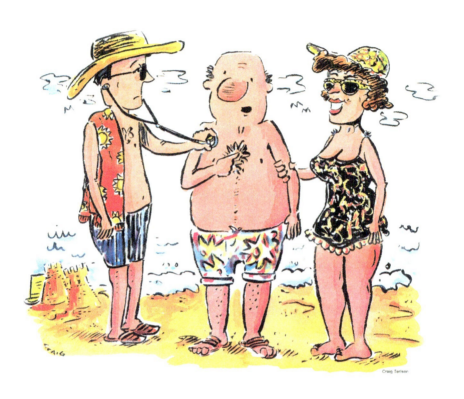

building. They did so, but evidently they missed me – too much as it turned out.

The wedding ceremony took place in the foyer and centre hall on the main floor of the building, and it was nearly over when Fay got off the elevator and spotted me. She did not seem to realize what was happening because, just as the bride whispered "I do," Fay said loudly, "Look who's here: my doctor!" The audience turned around to see me shushing this sweet lady. She quieted down and blushed red when she realized what was happening in her new home.

Not a minute later, hearing-impaired Sam made the same mistake. I guess I was sitting too close to the elevator. I tried to hide my face, but he had spotted me. Always effusive, Sam hobbled over and sat beside me. I tried to shush him, but that made him more expansive. Before I could stop him, he had me in a bear hug and said, "Good to see you, doc. What brings you here?" I pointed to the ceremony concluding in front of us, but Sam was also vision-impaired. He asked me several times, "What's going on?" as I tried to make myself invisible and as guests turned around to scold us.

Since then, our friends have married off their second daughter. Wisely, they held the wedding elsewhere. If they had held it in the same place, I'm not sure I'd have been invited.

Is there a doctor on the plane?

We were one hour into the three-hour flight from Florida to Toronto when the call came over the speaker system: "Is there a doctor aboard"? Without hesitation, I immediately identified myself.

At the time I had been watching the movie *High Anxiety* on the screen – a Mel Brooks classic about fear of heights. In the film he is the chief psychiatrist of the Hospital for the Very Very Nervous, yet he himself refuses to go on elevators and suffers from several other phobias, including an extreme fear of heights. The stage was set at 33,000 feet above sea level for the drama that followed.

I was directed to a young women suffering from severe chest pain and shortness of breath four rows behind me. The flight staff offered me the full emergency kit and the use of the galley, if I needed the patient to lie down. That was not essential because I am quite familiar with examining chests under clothing. I assured my patient she would not be embarrassed. All I needed was the stethoscope and blood-pressure cuff, but the stethoscope was useless against the roar of the plane's engines. Her pulse and her BP palpated at the wrist were normal.

Taking her history, I learned that she had experienced at least one panic attack and had been treated with antidepressant drugs in the past. I examined her legs for blood clots and found none, and she said she had not been on birth control drugs – a rare cause of clots and emboli. As we spoke her symptoms eased, and I informed the flight crew that an emergency landing was not necessary. To make sure, I sat beside her for the remaining one-and-a-half hours but wisely refrained from returning to my movie.

I was rewarded by relieved smiles from all the cabin staff and the captain as we left the plane. The patient was greeted by paramedics, who suggested a trip to Emergency at the closest hospital. She declined, and I could only hope I had not missed anything. To be on the safe side, I later contacted her family physician and then phoned her. All was well. Air Canada thanked me profusely and gave me enough air miles to get to the corner grocery store.

My only remaining dilemma is how to bill OHIP for an emergency plane call at 33,000 feet?

DOCTORS GET SICK TOO

Coronary heart disease

In 1991, at the age of fifty, I had open-heart surgery. It took me six years to disclose these personal facts about myself in the *Canadian Medical Association Journal*, prompted by the death of a colleague. Many things have happened in the lives of my family in the years since my cardio event, and I feel strongly that I should share my experience with others.

My genetic history was ominous: both of my parents had coronary heart disease. My father died at the age of seventy-three in 1989, outliving his mother by a generation with the help of antihypertensive drugs. He sustained a stroke, which led to his taking Aspirin, which led in turn to massive internal hemorrhaging and then a coronary – his one and only, despite his having disabling angina from the age of fifty on. Both his brothers have coronary disease. My mother had long-standing coronary disease and arrhythmia, but she outlived her brothers, all of whom smoked and died, respectively, at forty-two, forty-four, and fifty-four.

As I neared by fiftieth birthday, I took Oise, my Lhasa apso dog, for a walk one chilly October day and, while going uphill, I experienced severe chest pain. As soon as I stopped, the pain ceased. The diagnosis was easy: angina. My GP sent me for a stress test. It left me gasping for breath as a searing pain invaded my chest. The attending cardiologist was very interested in my ECG changes, forgetting momentarily that his patient was in great danger as the treadmill raced on up its own steep hill.

Twenty-five years before, in 1967, when I was an intern, two of our staff men had died on the table while having bypass surgery when it was in its infancy. I had been studying under a cardiology resident already known for his expertise, and I now called on him to perform my angiogram. His verdict? A 100 percent block in the heart's main artery, the left anterior descending, known as "the widow maker." There was also plaque damage in several other arteries. He recommended a six-vessel bypass operation.

On the day itself, a renowned cardiac surgeon took great pains as he diligently bypassed the six vessels. I woke the next day to find my wife and sons at my bedside. Apparently they had witnessed my violent hiccups, which can happen if the diaphragm is disturbed.

Post-op was smooth until two nurses knelt on either side of my bed and yanked out my four chest tubes. Warned that "this might hurt a bit," I shuddered as I felt that my innards were actually being dragged out in the process. But my surgeon was pleased, and he assured me I would not have problems for at least twenty years. I resumed my life after one week and went back to work after two months. I received great instruction on diet and exercise at the Toronto Cardiac Rehabilitation Centre once a week for six months, and I quit working evenings.

Ten uneventful years passed. My loving wife was spared widowhood. My sons thrived, and I was there to guide them. One became a psychiatrist, the other a capable businessman in the computer field.

❖ ❖ ❖

My local golf course has a hilly sixth hole that I had also sardonically called "the widow maker." After the drive sailed over the steep hill, I almost always found a way to climb that hill safely. But when this exertion left me panting for breath one day in 2000, I saw my cardiologist. He immediately arranged another angiogram.

This time the blockage was in a single artery that was amenable to stenting. The right coronary artery bypass had withered, but a lengthy stent was placed in the native artery, with great success. All the other 1991 arteries and veins were still wide open.

Eleven more years passed. Both my sons married – and, once the grandchildren began to arrive, they assured me of some immortality. My mother died at the age of eighty-six, not from her coronary disease but, like my father, from a gastrointestinal hemorrhage. Every one of her children and grandchildren was present, except for my brother's family in Israel. As we came into her room in intensive care, she asked, "Have you come to say goodbye?" They were her last words.

I tell my patients they can predict their future by close attention to their older siblings. My younger brother had a stroke at the age of fifty-five, from which he recovered. My younger sister watches her cholesterol intake and hopes to avoid this family problem. I quit working Fridays.

◈ ◈ ◈

On a cold windy night in April 2011, hurrying to a lecture at the University of Toronto, my wife and I had to walk too far in these trying conditions. The uphill stretch brought on significant chest pain and shortness of breath. I thought my twenty-year guarantee was up.

Once again I relied on my cardiologist's opinion of my vessels, and again the problem lay in my currently stented native right coronary artery. Five grandchildren had been born by then, so I certainly wanted to be around for another decade at least.

My interventional cardiologist placed a drug-eluting stent within my existing stent as I dozed. When I asked how far along he was, he said he was done. My bypassed vessels from 1991 looked good.

It is obvious that the only good thing about cardiovascular disease is that you can have it for a long time. I share this fact with my cardiac patients as we discuss their beta-blockers, blood thinners, ACE inhibitors, and statins. Like me, most of them have done very well, some for four decades or more.

I am now in my early seventies. Most physicians do not retire unless poor health intervenes, and I consider myself healthy. We generally slow down or semi-retire, and I am trying to accomplish this transition. It has been a great privilege to practise family medicine, and I won't hang up my white coat and stethoscope quite yet.

Sleep apnea

At great expense, some of my patients have purchased a made-to-order breathing device that now sits unused in a closet or is employed as a doorstop. I always encourage them to dust it off and try again: sleep apnea is a factor in heart disease, fatigue from lack of restful sleep, and car accidents caused by falling asleep at the wheel.

Sleep clinics have multiplied in recent years, to the detriment of our health budget: the investigation is expensive. Having participated in a few sleep studies myself, I have some important advice to pass on to colleagues and patients alike. Most important, when patients are released from this ordeal, without coffee or breakfast, often sleep-deprived and befuddled by the preceding night, they should not be driving. They should be picked up by a relative or friend at 6 a.m. to avoid accidents.

When physicians order a sleep study for a patient, they should be aware of the journey they are initiating. The test itself is an ordeal, and a positive result commits the hapless victim to a life on CPAP (continuous positive airwave pressure). As we know from our patients, this apparatus takes a lot of effort and discomfort to get accustomed to. My own experience has turned me into a masked spaceman, connected every night by a five-foot-long umbilical cord to a howling mothership quite capable of blowing my mind.

According to long-term complaints from my wife, my respiratory system, as I sleep, creates a high-volume cacophony of snorts, gasps, and choking sounds. Being sound asleep myself, I miss this performance, so for many a long year I ignored my better half. I could not, however, ignore my psychiatrist son, who confirmed my nocturnal adventures while we shared a room in Florida. When he added that there seemed to be rather long apneic periods as well, I decided it was time for a sleep study. My wife soon learned that the noises emanating from her spouse could get louder and even more bizarre during the "healing process."

On the night of my sleep study at the clinic, six other patients were booked, and I arrived just after a younger female patient. When the technician told us to follow her, I did so, right into the woman's bedroom instead of my own. Once informed that this facility was not that kind of place, I sheepishly entered my own room, where I noticed a closed-circuit camera and lots of electrical paraphernalia.

When I was in my pyjamas, the technician began a laborious process of attaching wires to my scalp, limbs, and torso, along with nose prongs for measuring oxygen and other things. All went well until she began to thread a wire under my pyjamas up my leg, to about mid-thigh but no higher. She asked me to reach under and pull the wire the rest of the way up, and it took me a while to understand her shyness to complete the job on her own.

By this time I was virtually immobilized by the cables, and one hand was occupied holding the battery. I was then asked to shuffle off to the washroom before settling down for the night. This task required careful aim, lest I short-circuit the system while voiding between the gear.

Once I was in bed, the technician went into her lab and, by intercom, told me in turn to shake a foot, a hand, and my head, then to move my eyes up and down and sideways, and finally to take a deep breath. Apparently I was wired correctly, so she said goodnight, telling me to beep her if my bladder needed emptying again during the next eight hours. There was no way I could even get through the door without her help, tied up as I was. The camera pointed at my bed made sure I was a good boy.

All I had to do was fall asleep and demonstrate my nocturnal theatrics – but I couldn't do it. I had been warned not to interfere with the important oxygen-level measuring lead attached to my index finger, and that required special effort with each change of position. The combination of a noisy ventilation system and the strange surroundings would not allow me to sleep, so I thought pleasant thoughts all night. I much appreciated the arrival of the technician to disconnect me at 6 a.m. and send me on my way. In my relief, I left my pyjamas on the bed.

What I thought was a sleepless night turned out to be a disturbed sleep with numerous awakenings. In technical language I had difficulty understanding, my respirologist described my sleep apnea and recommended a CPAP machine, starting at the low pressure and increasing. He sent me to our hospital's respiratory lab, where I met the young technician whose job it was to turn me into a perpetual spaceman. She tried me first with a nose mask, facilitated by a chinstrap to overcome any mouth-opening during the night – a phenomenon that causes the pressurized air to escape through the mouth. But the mask failed to do its duty, probably because my bald pate gave the strap no purchase.

And so I ended up with a full face mask. Now, the human face comes in many shapes, making it difficult to design a "one size fits all" mask. The very patient technician tried some fifteen different masks before she found the correct one to cover my nose and mouth. The mask must also allow for the various sideways head movements on the pillow. As an additional complication, the wearer is not supposed to sleep in the back position because the tongue tends then to drop back and cause obstruction.

During my attempts to sleep that first night, air escaped through several loose spots, causing a high-pitched whistle. I thought the popcorn-man of old was wheeling his trolley down my block. Then the entire machine fell onto the floor because I made a 360-degree turn, putting too much stress on the five-foot tubing. Of course, if the tubing had wound around my neck, worse things could have happened. After two or three more visits to the technician, I finally had a more successful seal. A repeat sleep study showed improvement in my oxygen levels. This time I remembered to take my pyjamas home.

The next step was to increase my air pressure from six centimetres to fourteen centimetres. This goal proved next to impossible to achieve, and air was forced out of my mask at several spots. The earlier whistle was nothing compared to this row. Once I thought a woodpecker had entered the mask, and another time I thought our home was being burglarized and our alarm was resounding off our walls. Every night became an adventure. Finally we compromised on a pressure I could handle, and I now use my equipment faithfully.

Before donning my mask, my bedtime ritual now involves putting a Band-Aid across the tip of my nose, lest a permanent groove develop there from the mask's pressure. Another problem is an inability to cuddle with my wife, lest we get tangled in the apparatus. She also receives annoying jets of air expelled through openings in the mask, necessary to avoid carbon monoxide poisoning. I must stay on good terms with her, because she could easily cover those grommets with her fingers while I sleep.

On one occasion she woke up, took a look at me, and screamed, forgetting that a spaceman was now occupying the other side of our bed. All I could think of to calm her down was to say, "Happy Mother's Day" – an appropriate comment that particular week. We exchanged glances, and several minutes of healing hysterical laughter followed.

BASEBALL as METAPHOR for the PRACTICE of MEDICINE

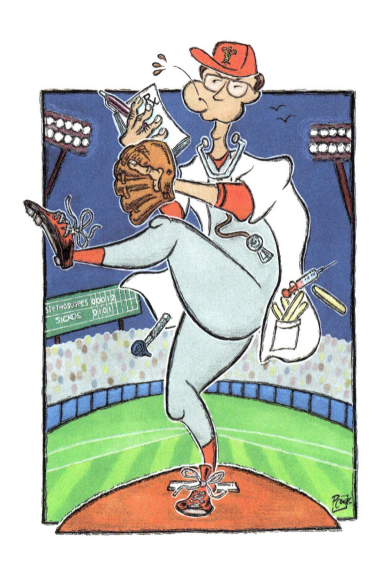

Doctors and baseball pitchers must get the opponent out

I like watching baseball on television. As I see some of the best pitchers sweating on the mound until they have retired the opposition batters, I often think that we physicians share the same defensive role, except that for us it's holding the line against disease. We perform in a game known as the doctor-patient relationship, some of which is just as confrontational as that of the pitcher-batter.

And so I sympathize with the baseball pitchers as they struggle to retire a difficult batter. Their opponents, like our worst patients, do the best they can to keep alive, fouling off the best pitches or, in our situation, adding new symptoms and complaints. Most patients are pleasant "easy-outs" to the experienced physician, but a few are impossible to retire gracefully with our composure still intact. In extreme cases, the patient may add a final insult, asking, "Is that all the time you have for me today?" To the physician, this question is perceived as the equivalent of the baseball batter thumbing his nose at the pitcher on his way around the bases after a hit.

That frustrated pitcher, high on his mound, may be yanked from the game by his manager if he fails, but physicians don't get off so easy, and our next few patients may suffer from our distress. There are many other similarities in the professional lives of a busy family physician and a baseball pitcher.

We face a similar number of challenges, more than twenty-five each day over a nine-hour period. The best baseball pitcher will need over a hundred pitches in total over nine innings to do his job. But if ten pitches are required in one player's at-bat, that leaves ninety pitches to retire all the others. Likewise, physicians cannot spend thirty or forty minutes with a single patient, allowing only ten or fifteen minutes each for the rest.

Before game-day, pitchers can study the records of every opposing batter. We also have a book on every patient that we can study before our day starts – the appointment book – and what a relief it is when we find no major challenges there. Some baseball pitchers and some physicians won't even look at this lineup in advance. Why get aggravated early?

Late in the game, pitchers are often called on to face "pinch hitters" – in medical parlance, extra patients needing to be seen, frequently at the end of a busy day. They can give big trouble to a tired doctor or pitcher. Only the pitcher, however, can get fresh relief from teammates in the bullpen.

Pitchers and physicians both work in front of a crowd whose mood can turn ugly: loyalty depends on performance. A full waiting room of delayed patients will hum, then grumble, and finally scold the secretary. We see and hear all this noise from our examining rooms and are very aware when patients have to wait too long. To us this buzz is the equivalent of baseball boos and jeers. A few disgusted patients will complain when they finally get up to bat, but it's unwise for participants to antagonize either of these professionals.

The pitcher can show his frustration with a batter by "brushing him back" with an inside pitch at high speed, causing him to reel back and fall in the dirt. Worse, he can bean the batter on his helmeted head or fracture one of his unprotected bones. Such retaliation is illegal, and he will be visited by umpires and face suspension.

Physicians have no desire to injure patients, but just as the canny pitcher can intimidate the batter and throw him off balance, we too can confound difficult patients by saying, "I am sorry, but we have only fifteen minutes today because I am overbooked." Physicians who are rude to patients generally regret their behaviour, especially if it leads to visits from officials and then suspension. Yelling must be avoided at all costs because inevitably it results in remorse.

Finally, comfortable retirement happens by the age of forty for most pitchers, but it is much later and often never in medicine. Our rewards lie in the daily gratitude most patients express, a constant ego-stroking that makes up for the heavy responsibilities we face with our neverending stream of patients.

When we occasionally save a patient's life or prevent a life of misery, the feeling of quiet inner happiness is impossible to describe. The baseball pitcher who has done a great job, who walks off the field tipping his hat to a thunderous standing ovation of 40,000 adoring fans, knows how we feel. Our patients quietly do the same for us.

A new seasonal affective disorder

The Toronto Blue Jays are making us sick. This new disorder is a variant of bipolar illness with addictive and obsessive-compulsive components as well.

My patient John was hopping mad last week at the overpaid and underachieving Toronto Blue Jays baseball team: they booted ground balls and blew a game with woeful hitting. During this tirade, he pushed his systolic blood pressure up thirty points and his pulse up by 50 percent. This reaction is bad news for any seventy-five-year-old, but it's not uncommon for many of my patients who feel they've been victimized by the game of professional baseball.

John was even more irritable because the extra innings had caused him to go to bed late, and then he slept poorly, visualizing the previous night's mistakes. Flushing red in the face, he concluded, "They should all drop dead!" Of course, if the Jays had ultimately won the game, all would have been forgiven, and John and I would have been glowing in praise of our athletic heroes. "How about those Blue Jays!"

It's odd: once the warm weather and sunshine arrives, just when we begin to feel better, in comes this new weather-related ailment. Like so many Canadian fans, my mood rises and falls with the success of the Jays from April to October. After a busy workday, my leisure activity is dominated fully six days a week at home or in the SkyDome in three- to five-hour shifts, for 162 games a year – and more if by chance they make the playoffs.

I watch in my "man-cave," living a separate life from my wife in the family room. While she leads a normal life chatting with friends, my emotions are on a roller coaster. Occasionally she pads into my

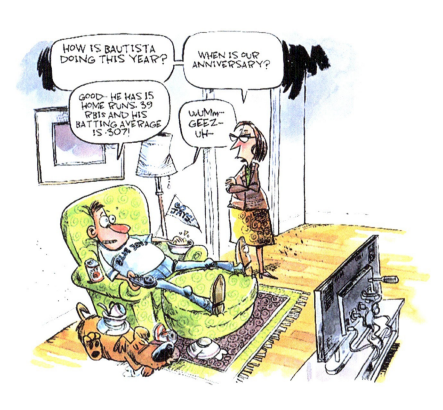

A new seasonal affective disorder

room to see what the yelling is all about and to make sure I'm not having a seizure or apoplexy.

I believe that negative experiences following a professional baseball team are common enough to warrant a separate entry in the Diagnostic and Statistical Manual, the psychiatric game book, as a bipolar illness with an addictive component. Consider the evidence: although baseball is considered by many to be the most boring game on earth, true devotees cannot miss a single inning, not even the pre-game and post-game shows. This addiction means that all useful work is put aside on most weeknights and weekend afternoons. Socializing is done by phone between innings, while romance must wait for the exhausted, nerve-jangled, and bug-eyed fans to catch their breath. Canadians cannot escape the game even if they are out strolling or walking the dog because there is a constant buzz on patio radios of commentators doing the play-by-play.

The addictive nature of this illness became obvious to me after a rare evening out when I could not get the game results fast enough on arriving home at eleven o'clock at night. TV news programs coyly tease fans by withholding sports until the end of the news hour, and by this time I was pale and sweaty and tremulous, badly missing my "fix."

Far worse, during the baseball strike of 1994 we were cut off abruptly and completely. This acute withdrawal left me with insomnia, caused by nightmares of curve balls aimed at my head. I was irritable and less responsive to a large influx of patients with the same symptoms. Then I realized that most of them were also suffering from the "baseball blues," and we soon began to practise group therapy on each other.

It is obvious that we bipolar baseball fans had better lighten up. Our emotional happiness must not depend on an umpire's faulty eyesight, opponents stealing our bases, and our own relief pitcher's inopportune wildness followed by a beefy opponent hitting the ball over the outfield fence.

The only solution is to gradually reduce our baseball addiction the same way patients are taken off an addictive drug – watching one game less per week until we are off it completely or down to a manageable level of one or two contests per week. We must go to sleep hungry, as it were, for the game results. Our local morning newspapers must satisfy us the next day, after a far more restful sleep.

BODY IMAGE and PLASTIC SURGERY

The widow's facelift

As a family physician I am occasionally asked about facelifts, but I was truly surprised when a seventy-year-old woman raised this subject. Many patients discuss facelifts in a casual manner, merely seeking information. Mary, however, was quite serious.

Mary was sixty years old when she and her second husband became my patients. In retrospect I realize I should have inquired about the reason for her first husband's death because it soon became apparent that she went through men quickly. Mary was a plain-looking woman, yet she turned out to be a champion in the highly competitive field of finding a husband at this time of life. Each of her unions was duly and promptly sanctified. Time was of the essence, as her story later proved.

Husband no. 2 was much older than Mary, and he did not last long before succumbing to heart disease. Mary was a very attentive wife to him in his final illness, and at this point I had no reason to suspect her of any misdeeds. Over the next few years, however, two more frail and older husbands came and went. When they were well enough to accompany her to my office, they appeared to be far into Shakespeare's last act. One was wheelchair-bound; the other had an oxygen tank. Strangely, neither man ever became my patient, but Mary told me quite a lot about them, placing herself in the martyr's role. Sick old men are not easy to look after. Besides all Mary's housekeeping and nursing duties, she had numerous doctors to visit and medical tests to arrange for her husbands as well as frequent hospital admissions. Mary had to master complicated drug regimens and prepare special meals to suit some of their illnesses. Unfortunately, harmful "mistakes" can occur at any stage, with little chance of discovery.

After husband no. 4 had died, Mary asked me to arrange facelift surgery. When I inquired why she wanted this operation, she replied that it would improve her marriageability and consequent financial security. She said she was still rather impoverished and needed support to live well and in a nice home. I discouraged Mary from having this cosmetic surgery because of her age and her heart disease. She must have noticed some surprise or amusement in my response, because she left my practice soon after. Perhaps she felt I knew too much. I never saw her again, or perhaps I did, without recognizing her new face.

Mary wasn't "lost to follow-up," however. Several years later, when I was chatting with her cardiologist, he told me that after her facelift, Mary met husband no. 5 and now winters in Florida in his condominium. My colleague also told me the secret of Mary's repeated successes: she responded to men's entreaties in the personal columns of local newspapers and, to guarantee interest, included the picture of a beautiful and somewhat younger woman. Once the man met her, her personality did the rest.

Her method failed at least once. A retired military man, obviously with better vision than the rest, had kept right on marching when she greeted him with outstretched hand at their "rendezvous" point. Mary is an example of a poor marriage risk but an excellent opportunist in the game of love.

Why plastic surgery patients switch doctors

Some colleagues and I have discovered an almost sure way to inadvertently lose patients. When people opt for plastic surgery they seem to become extremely sensitive and self-conscious, and it's all too easy for them to interpret perfectly innocent comments as insensitive intrusions on their privacy. Here are a few examples garnered over many years as a family physician.

> BREASTS: Twenty years ago, a slim twenty-year-old patient insisted on breast augmentation, and I tried unsuccessfully to discourage her. She left my practice soon after the surgery, but I saw her recently when she came to talk to me about her mother. Today we are aware of many silicone problems, including potential disease, so I was curious to hear her thoughts on this procedure now. She said she would like to have her implants replaced, though that seemed unwise to me. In the last several years, smaller breasts have been more acceptable, and fewer women undergo augmentation. Rather, they request breast reductions. Large breasts can be very heavy, moreover, and lead to back problems. I assisted on one reduction surgery and can testify that it is a very bloody and crude business, though well worth it. My one concern about breast surgery is that it may make the future interpretation of mammograms more difficult.
>
> NOSE: Plastic surgery can work astounding changes in this area. A long-term patient came to see me after a rhinoplasty, and I didn't know who she was. This operation was done after a personal tragedy, when she was likely making an

effort to start afresh, but for some reason she also left me for a different doctor. Another young woman in my practice had a bad result. It was difficult for me to maintain my dignity as I looked clinically at her nose tip, which was pointing off to one side. Her next mistake was accepting a "free" repair by the same surgeon. A second plastic surgeon finally put her face together properly. When I last heard from her, just before she moved to another city, she was considering a "tummy tuck."

In our zeal to be helpful, family physicians can make errors in judgment. One teenage boy with a huge nose was not offended when I told him to consider surgery. He responded that his nose looked fine to him. Yet he also fired me, but about ten years later, when this incident I thought was forgotten. I have another male patient, age around fifty, whose nose desperately needs doing, but I have kept my big mouth shut. Still, I have an overpowering urge to recommend a nose fix.

FACELIFT: When a fifty-five-year-old lady saw me for the first time, I couldn't believe how young she looked until I saw the telltale scars behind her ears. This surgery took at least five years off her face. And one of my friends had a very successful transformation at the age of seventy-five but died two years later. If you're contemplating this procedure, don't wait too long.

HAIR: Several men have undergone hair transplants, with generally poor results. One thirty-year-old quit my practice after I said, quite innocently, that his scalp and hair distribution made his tresses resemble the head of a doll, especially on windy days.

PENIS: Several men had plastic inserts for impotence in the 1990s. I assisted at one of these procedures, helping with the placement of a boomerang-shaped rod, half in the body and half in the shaft of the penis. These men ended up with permanent erections, which could be hidden by clothing or by strapping the penis to the belly, but they have to be wary in a health club's communal shower room, in case they come under suspicion. To this day I am shocked when faced with an erection during physical examinations because men do not get erections during checkups. In these cases the penis literally pops up like a jack-in-the-box as soon as I pull the underwear down. In recent years, Viagra has largely eliminated the need for this surgery.

Colleagues agree with me that they also lose some of their patients after they have undergone plastic surgery. In addition to the usual reasons of self-consciousness and the wish for new beginnings, perhaps these people are by nature more adventurous, so they find it easy to find multiple reasons to switch their doctors. Whatever the logic, it seems that the physician must exercise considerable kindness and discretion – and in recent years I've scored much better with this group of patients than I used to do.

In my opinion, there are three simple ways to look better:

- A wig can shave at least a decade off the appearance of some elderly women. They age incredibly when the wig comes off, as when they are lying down flat on their backs or pulling a sweater over their heads. Generally their own hair is sparse and untended, and I have to be very careful not to let the surprise at their rapid aging show on my face.
- Even the most beautiful woman looks studious and ordinary with eyeglasses on. For those who are really interested in their appearance, it's better to deceive the world as my mother did,

while engaged to my father. As she later confessed, every movie they saw together at that time was a blur. Contact lenses are a better idea.

- Along with regular dental care, orthodonture creates an invaluable nice smile. Several adult patients have benefited from my advice in this regard.

As for me, my sparse head hair is a problem only to my teasing son, not to me. Orthodonture was helpful, but when my cousin saw my braces, she asked, "So, when are you getting a nose job?" Never, so far, but in a weak moment I did ask my plastic surgeon friend about a chin implant. He pointed out that I did not need it because the problem disappeared when I smiled. Since then I have kept on smiling.

My nude dye job

Vanity won out. After years of resistance, I finally accepted the fact that I might look better with my original brown hair colour. The grey melted away – not at the hands of my barber, who, anticipating a big monthly payoff, had treated me to a sample. No, it was my wife who offered to do the job, and I can now describe the somewhat hysterical procedure that takes place when folks attempt a dye job at home.

I suspect that many wives would be happy to engage in such grooming behaviour if their husbands agreed. The transformation is best performed with both parties nearly nude, because the dye is lethal on clothes. With me sitting on a low bench, my wife gloved herself and mixed her brew – a great improvement over Grecian Formula and similar products, she said. She then assumed a rather dangerous position before my person and applied the chemical with a brush.

The temptation to tickle had to be resisted: if the dye winds up on your forehead or nose, it will stay there for some time. There were, however, many giggle-producing comments from each of us, which threatened her steady hand. Of course, most men needing this dye job will have been married long enough to keep their libidos in check, at least temporarily.

Once the lathering was done, I had to sit quietly and alone for twenty minutes as the magic transformation took place. I could have read, but it was difficult because the dye itched and I dared not scratch. I was desperate to rinse the goo off, shampoo and shower vigorously, and towel off and rest for a bit.

The results of our first attempt were pleasing, and many patients commented on my youthful appearance. My response? "Only my wife knows for sure." The cost and time involved were trivial compared to a salon treatment. And the opportunities for bonding were priceless.

The obvious question is whether I (or most men) can be trusted to return the favour for our wives. Most women have myriad excuses to avoid the experiment: we're too sloppy, too tempted to wander geographically; and they're too scared to risk sitting in this vulnerable condition before a potential tickler. Besides, most spouses have a glorious abundance of hair, and it would be a shame for it to appear mottled or multicoloured after an amateur dye job. I suspect most women will opt to leave the whole process to the professionals.

Bald and balder – or a tale of two drug reps

You get a bit paranoid when you are chatting with a drug rep and he seems to be sneaking a peek at your head and, more specifically, at your hair distribution. But that happened about ten years ago now, and I had reasons to find this behaviour acceptable at the time.

No doubt this Rogaine brand rep was surveying the territory in question because he felt that his minoxidil had a better chance of a happy greeting from the less hirsute docs on his route. He certainly got the royal treatment from me. Although I had patients waiting when he arrived, I took a look at his heavy briefcase and told my secretary to show him in.

We shook hands, and I listened intently as he began to detail me about minoxidil – facts I already knew from journal ads and the media campaign in bus shelters and on television. Could he be my own saviour? Did he really have the goods in his briefcase?

He asked me diplomatically if I would like a sample for personal use. It must surely be awkward to tell a physician that the nakedness of his head is obvious. Noting my breathless eagerness, the rep pulled out a bottle and passed it to me. I signed his form and bade him goodbye, all the while clutching the bottle in my lab-coat pocket. He promised another month's supply at his next visit.

By now at mid-morning there were several patients in my waiting room. Regardless, I just had to open that precious bottle and give it a try, so I smeared some of the liquid onto my scalp. I made the cardinal error common to men: I began this project without reading the directions. Once I finished with my patients, I spent the lunch hour looking up the potential adverse reactions to Rogaine in my drug manual.

Being a confirmed hypochondriac at the time, I knew by the end of the first paragraph that minoxidil was not for me. After my single dose, my high anxiety level had already given me most of the rare symptoms described in the next few paragraphs, including flushing, dizziness, shortness of breath, and a rapid heart rate.

After a month, when the Rogaine rep reappeared with another bottle, I politely declined his generous offer. My personal experience, however, had not prevented me from carefully prescribing minoxidil to my patients, with some positive results.

A decade went by, by which time I was reconciled to having a "low-maintenance pate." My barber calls me "the Ten-Minute Man" because he never has trouble fitting me into his schedule – at full price, of course.

A man sees things quite differently as a fifty-something, when other changes have occurred in his body. Grey hair means that you appear as a hairless phantom in family pictures anyway, particularly if your spouse colours her hair. How's that for a rationalization?

Enter a second pharmaceutical representative, this time an attractive young woman, to spoil my contentment. I call her Propecia Patty. The drug she was promoting was "finasteride 1 mg," a competitor to minoxidil. This oral medication had arrived as a hair product via a circuitous route through the urinary tract. A patient on Proscar 5 mg, the same finasteride but in a bigger dosage for prostate problems, had done some reading and had paved the way for this alternative therapy when he showed some new hair growth.

Once in my office, the comely rep also gave my scalp a few surreptitious glances, but women are better at concealing these things than are men. With the enthusiasm common to all members of her profession, she invited me to an endocrinologist's talk on this subject in a fine hotel. Then, wearing her scientist hat, she told me how research done on pseudohermaphrodites had led to the hair-raising discovery of her drug's abilities.

But this remedy wasn't for me. As Propecia Patty spoke, I silently prided myself that baldness is a sign of virility, perhaps due to an extra dollop of circulating testosterone, a hormone quite a few men my age are now happy to pay for because of so-called andropause. Yet another rationalization!

As most physicians know, coincidences occur frequently in the practice of medicine. If the Rogaine rep and Propecia Patty show up in my waiting room at the same time, I will invite them in to debate the merits of their competing products, with me as referee should the discussion get too hot.

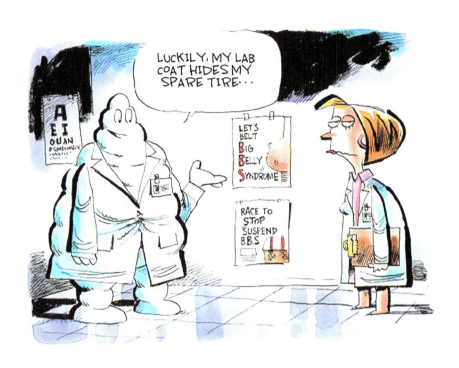

Big-belly syndrome

Gravity and gluttony have created an uncomfortable problem for me and some of my senior male colleagues. One old friend scared me as he opened his lab coat and approached me in the corridor of our clinic at a very high speed. He had an obvious intent to do the belly bounce, and his was much bigger than mine. I sidestepped like a matador and escaped injury.

This experience got me thinking creatively. At the next major medical conference I attended, I found that "big-belly syndrome" (BBS) was much in evidence. Every time I tried to shake hands with an older friend, we bounced off each other. A hug was out of the question because our arms were simply not long enough.

The growth of your belly can be read as easily as tree rings by a close look at the notches on your favourite belt. Most physicians know that when some men buy a belt, they think it lasts forever. Those notches are very telling, so if you are one of these culprits, just buy a new and longer belt.

To hide what appears to be a nine-month pregnancy, it is possible to look wise, while standing, by crossing our arms and resting them on this "anatomical armrest." We can also do a fair job in our offices by simply buttoning up our white lab coats. I have always maintained that lab coats cover any number of sartorial and physical sins.

You know you are on the way to BBS if you can no longer see your feet while standing. When you drip gravy or ice cream, it no longer hits the floor. Trousers get tighter at the waist until, finally, you wear the belt below the belly, even if you also have suspenders. On one occasion I tried not wearing a belt. That led to my trousers slowly slipping down a few inches and threatening to go all the way.

My lab coat hid this embarrassment, but I could not adjust myself while standing and talking to a female patient. I sat down until she left.

Men of our age are at a urinary disadvantage, with prostatic problems leading to frequent visits to the washroom. With BBS, when standing to void, the penis finally disappears below the overhanging belly. That creates a directional problem. Basically, if you don't hear a tinkle, you are probably peeing on your shoes. Children are honest, and one five-year-old boy, on seeing his ample father in the shower, announced, "Mommy, Daddy doesn't have a penis!"

My biggest patient, John, has a belly measuring sixty-two inches. He can barely get through my doors. At his last visit, when I called him in, he found he was stuck in my waiting-room armchair. He needed the help of several other patients, some tugging and some holding until he extricated his huge hips. John has to pay for two seats on airplanes and is very unpopular on buses and in movie theatres.

Surgery to remove the fatty apron is ill-advised. When making rounds one day I bumped into the plastic surgeon to whom I have referred many patients over the years. "Steve," I begged, while pointing down at the area in question, "Can you do anything about my spare tire?" He staggered away laughing so loud that he had tears in his eyes. I took that as a no, but I continue to send patients to him.

I have one demanding patient who, in his fifties, insisted that I find him a surgeon willing to cut a few inches from his abdominal fat. He was left with drainage complications for months until the surgeon agreed to repair the mess at no expense. In my experience, any time a surgeon repairs things gratis, he is embarrassed about the first result. My patient is certainly more svelte now but just as tiresome.

Liposuction is done in a few private offices in Toronto, but some hopeful patients have had complications, and there have been a few deaths as a result of incompetence and neglect. I would rather be fat. Bariatric surgery to shrink the stomach and shorten the intestines is also risky, and even a marked weight loss does not always reduce BBS. Again, stay fat.

SEX

Fleeing from temptation

Family physicians often chat with patients about current events, and several years ago now I was interested in what my patients had to say about American president Bill Clinton's problems with Monica Lewinsky, the young White House intern with whom he had a lengthy affair. There are profound implications in this story, at least for male physicians who might become sexually involved with patients.

On a lighter note, most of my elderly patients are confused about the term "oral sex." They think it has something to do with talking or kissing. And few can figure out what the president's cigars had to do with sex unless he smoked one after each tryst. They are equally puzzled about why anyone would want to test a stain on any of their dresses for DNA, thinking of soup splotches or mustard residue.

The women tend to blame Monica, saying she was a flirt who had no business taking a married man aside to show him her underwear. The men are a bit wiser (not much), and they blame the president. He took advantage of an easy situation, they say, because he has no "stop button" on his libido.

In the medical world, such taboo situations develop in one of three ways: the doctor is seductive, the patient is seductive, or there is a combination of both. We read about sexually abusive physicians in Ontario every time the College of Physicians and Surgeons publishes its list of those (mostly men) charged, after a prolonged investigation, with sexual assault on one or more patients, usually female. This charge often brings a sad end to an otherwise exemplary career, with the accused feeling shame every time he greets a colleague. Bad news travels fast.

Every innocent male physician is an authority figure, and as such he may become a target or a trophy for susceptible women in the course of his work. He must literally run from these pursuers: they may become bolder with each visit, wearing revealing clothing and suggestive smiles though tons of makeup. The doc should not be flattered, because this behaviour probably happens as much to us ordinary joes as it happens to those who think highly of their looks and manner. Rather, he should remember that our disciplinary body has zero-tolerance for those who stray.

One formerly esteemed colleague was allowed to end his career by retiring after several patients detailed his fondness for breast exams, which were totally unnecessary in his specialty. In another case, a patient attended group therapy for years until it was discovered that the psychiatrist in charge was choosing women in the class to seduce. One inventive pediatrician selected from the anxious mothers of his patients, while a geriatrician found his victims among the anxious daughters of his patients. Female physicians are also tempted and may succumb, in one case after inviting a male patient to a nightclub for drinking and dancing, then to her condo for further "counselling."

Before offering preventive techniques I have learned over many years, I should state that, at this stage in my career, I have little temptation in my own office: my patients have aged along with me and are now mainly quite old. I do sometimes exit an examining room flushed and smeared with lipstick and reeking of perfume, but that is only because I was unable to dodge the thankful but determined embrace of a granny.

At the first sign of trouble, a no-nonsense professional manner may disarm the patient wielding Cupid's bow. If not, we should keep the visits brief and invite the nurse in before doing physical examinations of any kind.

My advice to colleagues and to Bill Clinton: Just say no!

Viagra – making sex fun at any age

The important subject of sexual relations is almost never discussed by female patients with male physicians, but I suspect their husbands have been encouraged to have "the talk." The men speak up only after their wives have left the room. Before Viagra, all I could offer was penile injections and other suspect remedies.

An entire subculture has developed in the years since Viagra was introduced, followed by Cialis and Levitra. I prescribe them all. Their ads are ubiquitous, especially at sporting events, but *Maclean's* magazine has also featured these products in a front-cover article. These ads are aimed mainly at the age forty to seventy demographic, both male and female, with the women expected to prod their mates along to the family physician and the drugstore.

Most of us have seen the television commercial in which men and women prance out of their homes and frolic in the street to the music of "We are the Champions." Many different target groups are represented among these Viagrans, including the wheelchair-bound, women, blacks, the obese, nerds, the elderly, and even postal workers. Taken together, they cover a lot of territory and seem to illustrate that all these folks have been having great sex.

In one Cialis ad, a couple race around frantically with smiles and knowing looks on their faces as they handle neglected household emergencies. The smoke detector is screaming and the dog is howling. During their spontaneous moment of passion, the tub has overflowed, the roast in the oven has burned, and their dog, desperately scratching to go out, has messed the floor. Cialis now sponsors a golf tournament.

Here are some subgroups I have successfully treated as a family physician. Details have been altered to protect identities, but rest assured we hear it all.

The recreational Viagran is the youngest in the group and really quite potent without my help. His efforts to improve on perfection may lead to embarrassing trips to hospitals with an erection that won't go down. He may actually mix Viagra with illicit drugs at party time. At this age the pill can be tried for premature ejaculation with some success.

The mid-life Viagran, if depressed, may have been rendered happier but impotent by one of several modern antidepressant drugs. He may respond well. One man in his forties prefers Cialis, the "weekender," which renders him potent for thirty-six hours. With eager anticipation he takes it Friday night. Even if he argues with his wife on Saturday, he is still available for great "make-up" sex on Sunday.

The philanderer Viagran is usually past the age of fifty, and his unaccustomed ability may exceed his wife's tolerance level. His zeal may entice him to go elsewhere. Some rogues say they need Viagra only when they are with their wives, never when with a girlfriend. They insist on a separate prescription for Viagra, which they fill at a pharmacy far from home. If a wife ever discovers these purchases, these guys have some explaining to do. The drug did not make them unfaithful; it merely makes their cheating more fun. We family physicians know about infidelity because we treat the subsequent STDs.

The suicidal Viagran by age sixty may have developed coronary heart disease or prostate disease. He may be a risk-taker, because Viagra may conflict with his current drugs and cause his death from low blood pressure. The cardiac patient feels sex is worth it, so he simply skips his nitrate drugs on those days. The prostate sufferer skips his alpha-blockers if he expects to get lucky. Afterward, these guys may be found sitting beside each other in a hospital emergency room, one with a coronary, and his neighbour with a distended bladder that won't empty.

The old-old Viagran, if widowed, may find a younger girlfriend who tells him, "Every intimate relationship between a man and a woman should include sex. Ask your doctor for those pills we see advertised on TV." After a discussion with one such patient, he replied: "Doc, no way am I taking that chance. She'll have to be satisfied with a cuddle. I know I am." She wasn't.

PARENTS
and
ELDERLY
PATIENTS

My parents – our waiting-room spies

When my mother appeared in our waiting room, everything got lively, heralded by the buzz of conversation I soon heard from my consulting room. Her visits could be a major factor in my office because she often arrived an hour early for transportation reasons and had to stay long after she was seen by Dr. Susan, my associate. Instead of coming into the inner office, she preferred to sit where the action was. While waiting to be seen, she had the ability to charm her ever-changing audience as patients came and went. She got female patients to chat by her friendly smile and compliments about their hairstyles. With older men, she simply asked which doctor they were seeing, and then asked probing questions if they were seeing me.

Despite my pleas, Mom insisted on telling the other patients who she was, once she had concluded her interview. Predictably, she then became an instant celebrity. My patients inevitably told her how wonderful I was. None would dare say anything negative about me: although she was short, she was feisty – and on home territory, so to speak. In turn, many patients had nice things to tell me later about my mother. Really, though, what fool of a patient could criticize the doctor's mother to his face? Only those with a death-wish need apply.

As a bonus, mother discussed their various health problems, if time permitted, and had an opinion about any ailment yet discovered. She gained the confidence of others by revealing her own ailments and happily joined in conversations about treatments. One man even said he could leave without seeing me because Mom had set his complaint in order. She speedily convinced him to linger, saying, "Oh no, please don't leave, my son will get annoyed with me."

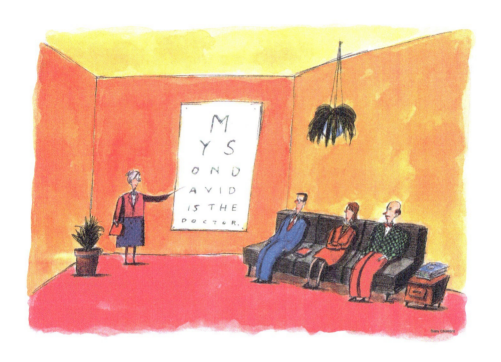

As it turned out, the man in question might have done better listening to Mom, but he survived anyway.

On those days when Mom preferred to stay anonymous, her detective work was simplicity itself. Her side of the conversation went this way:

"Whose patient are you?" (She does not carry on this way with my associate's patients.)

"For how many years?"

"Does he ever talk about his mother?"

"Do you like his care?"

"Do you think that the office runs well?"

"How about the secretarial staff?"

(Again) "Does he ever talk about his mother?"

When we finally got to say hello, Mom told me the results of her investigation and revealed which patients were dissatisfied. I also found out who was crabby about a long wait or who made disparaging grumbles as they left, oblivious to the little secret agent in the corner. Mom was smart enough to steer clear of the more taciturn patients and those who appeared disturbed or peculiar. Every physician has some of these types. Later, when she was debriefed, I got the benefit of her motherly advice about which patient I should be careful with or even "fire" as soon as possible from my practice. "Lose that guy, he is a real psycho," she'd say, or "That sneezing woman is full of germs; put on a mask when you see her."

One day she spotted a young female patient of the sort that can be hazardous to male physicians. She was dressed and made-up seductively, and in short order Mom learned that she worked in a massage parlour and had found me cute on an earlier visit. As a preventive measure, Mom interrupted me with this news before I even saw the woman, so I kept a staff person in the room during my examination.

To my surprise and embarrassment, Mom carried on her celebrity routine even when she was admitted to my hospital. She informed the entire nursing staff and many of my colleagues of my brilliance and superb clinical skills. By coincidence, she once had a hospital roommate who was my patient, so a lot was said in the few days they were together. Their proximity even led to a great compliment for my mother, who was indeed quite youthful looking. My elderly and somewhat near-sighted patient thought she was my wife. I did not tell Mom about this flattering statement for a while, saving it for the right occasion, to be used as ammunition in the ongoing political strife common to any extended family. Of course, Mom delighted in relating this story to her friends – over and over again.

Besides raising four children and working alongside Dad in their grocery store, often with babe in arms, Mom had found time to care for her own parents and her in-laws. The close association among all our families gave me my earliest medical knowledge as they went from stroke to diabetes to coronary heart disease to brain tumour to colon cancer, and from hospital to nursing home and, finally, to the death of the previous generation. I was lucky enough to have grandparents until my teens, and Mom was there for them all.

Lest the reader think my story is unique, I discovered that Mom did a similar routine when she was visiting the offices of other doctors and dentists in our family. She could not keep her pride a secret, so she expressed her feelings openly in all her public relations. These promotions did no harm, of course; they kept her busy, and she loved it!

Mom died suddenly in 2008 at the age of eighty-five, after suffering an internal hemorrhage. She had lived long enough to be a major influence on her grandchildren, and all but three of her children and grandchildren were present that day. We phoned my brother and his sons in Israel, and he spoke to her. We like to think that she heard him. My esteemed surgical colleague told us there was no hope, and she died six hours later. The elder of my two sisters knew that she herself would soon die of ovarian cancer that horrible year. I am sure that if my sister had died first, Mom would have been a tower of strength in her daughter's last four months. At least she was spared the ordeal of burying a child.

I cannot leave this story without detailing my father's role. He was the one who gave me the confidence to apply to medical school, and his many maladies and his treating physicians were also influential in my career. Dad lived for seventy-three years, but they were not enough. As a firstborn son during the Depression, he struggled to help his parents in their grocery store. Seeing how hard they all worked for eighteen hours a day, he rebelled and missed a golden opportunity to become a pharmacist, balking at those brutal hours. He had endured enough of this routine, he thought. A few years later, however, he wound up the same way anyhow – a grocer.

After he left the Air Force, the Canadian government would have subsidized his education, but he turned this offer down, condemning himself to a series of tough jobs interspersed with yet another grocery store every time he quit. This itinerant life meant a lot of dislocation for us kids: although we stayed in the Toronto area, each district then was a village unto itself. He worked at various times for the post office and a real estate company, as a chauffeur and a parking-lot attendant. In his prime, he was employed by two dairies, but in his senior years he had an office job at City Hall.

As professionals, we physicians may forget the respect and privileges we enjoy in being the masters of our own fate. The difference in lifestyle between a professional person and a worker is enormous. Dad's younger brothers, with the same intelligence, became leaders in their professions. Dad missed out, but he and Mom made sure that all their own children went to university and reached their potential.

Meantime, my mother gave birth every few years, and, as I am also a firstborn, I remember well the pride in his eyes when he and my mother brought Larry, then Nora, and finally Susie home from the hospital. Every time he expressed his pleasure by saying: "We may be poor, Rosie, but this child makes us millionaires. There is nothing more we need." A fourth child to a family struggling financially was a surprise, but in a few years it was the sight of Susie bounding down the path into his arms at day's end that made him forget work for a while.

My father was a man who could never understand why he kept getting sick, despite all the doctors in his family. His brother, son, daughter, and son-in-law should have ensured his good health forever, in his opinion. But the passing years brought more and more ill health. Despite our collective medical incompetence where he was concerned, Dad swelled with pride at our profession. Like most people, he held physicians in the highest regard – no doubt in part from his trying to afford medical care for his wife and four children on a working man's salary. None of us suffered, but we certainly saw doctors very seldom compared to current routines.

Dad was never one to suffer in silence, and he promptly had four conflicting medical opinions from his family about each new symptom. And, while many patients are non-compliant, he was a man who never missed a pill. He told us often about his "pill count" – thirty-five daily at the end. For twenty-five years medications for angina pectoris kept him going, but with many side effects.

My father was seldom well, and through taking him to many of his doctor appointments over the years, I witnessed medical care at its best – unhurried history taking and thorough examination, followed by wise advice. In his last illness, I marvelled at the skill of his critical-care physicians and at the dedication of the surgeon who operated on Dad at four in the morning.

When it was all over, we kids were surprised that Dad had saved enough over the years to allow my mother to live well and independently. It should not have been a surprise, for it was the product of meagre earnings and self-denial. It was all part of the immigrant experience, so common to the brave souls who came to Canada from different parts of the world.

Dad was largely responsible for my career choice. He pointed out that doctors are never unemployed – an important point for him because he had been through a brief episode of demoralizing unemployment. The expression "My son the doctor" was always very meaningful for both my parents, but a bit of a joke for me until one of my own sons was accepted into medical school. Medicine remains one of the most respected professions, a guarantee that your child will have a rewarding and enjoyable career.

Whenever I visit my parents' graves, I picture them on their front porch, smiling hello and waving goodbye. The loss of a parent is devastating, after we have taken them for granted for so many years. My advice to readers: Jump in your car, visit your parents, and give them a big hug. If they wonder about this show of affection, tell them I sent you.

I will never forget Dad's last words to me: "Look after your mother. She's a good woman."

Death takes a holiday

I am delighted to report on a phenomenon I have recently detected in my practice of medicine among the elderly: people have stopped dying. Now, I know this happy situation can't possibly last because that would be against the laws of nature. Still, for the time being, my patients seem to be coasting along in fine fettle, whistling past the disasters they have avoided or may never have to face.

Many of them are old now: hundreds are over the age of 75, and quite a few are over the age of 90. The oldest, at 102, has just begun computer lessons and is threatening to join a folk-dancing class once I strengthen his bones. They faithfully keep their appointments and follow the medical advice they receive. Preventive medicine, distaste for smoking, and regular exercise have helped, with luck thrown in for good measure.

The reasons for this success are quite simple: regular checkups, including prostate and pelvic examinations; simple but timely lab work often costing only a few dollars; astute attention to signs and symptoms well known to patients and physicians; and the use of medications – some quite inexpensive and ancient, some quite costly.

Heart disease, stroke, and cancer are the three big killers, but they have become strangely silent among my patients, to the delight of all concerned. We will never eliminate coronary heart disease without a drastic change in diet and lifestyle. Yet very few patients these days go on to have an actual coronary thrombosis provided they and their physicians pay attention to the very simple symptoms of angina.

Most patients can throw out their nitroglycerin bottles if the usual investigations lead to the correction of narrowed arteries by medications, stenting/angioplasty, or, in the last resort, coronary artery bypass grafting. More than a hundred of my patients, friends, and colleagues, myself included, are long-term survivors of this wonderful procedure.

What about strokes? It must be obvious to anyone who is observant that today we encounter far fewer stroke-disabled persons than in times past. There are three reasons for this change: control of high blood pressure with an array of easily tolerated drugs from several classes; control of irregular heartbeat, at times by a pacemaker, together with blood thinners to prevent blood clots; and close attention to the warning signs. A "completed stroke" is almost as rare as a completed coronary thrombosis.

Coated Aspirin remains the most commonly used blood thinner, while lipid-lowering drugs, statins, and fibrates seem almost to dissolve arterial plaque. That is not actually possible, but these drugs work as if they did, with great benefits in coronary and stroke prevention.

Cancer comes in many deadly forms, but most can be thwarted through luck and intelligence – it's still all about attention paid to early warnings. Mercifully, none of my elderly patients have died from breast cancer in well over five years. The last two victims were guilty of ignoring obvious masses, fearful of seeking medical attention until it was too late. Is there a debate about mammography in my world? Certainly not. About fifteen of my current patients are alive many years later because of it. Some have forgotten that they ever had breast cancer.

Uterine and cervical cancer yield easily to regular examination and attention to unusual bleeding; ovarian cancer remains the most difficult woman's cancer to detect, but timely ultrasound is invaluable.

Colon cancer if neglected has a terrible death rate. But colonoscopy done for positive family history, or for anemia, bleeding, pain, or a change in bowel habits can lead to a complete cure while the cancer is harmlessly confined to a polyp. Stomach cancer is heralded by anemia and by black stool, and is likewise treatable if caught early. Elderly persons merit a hemoglobin every six months to detect the anemia of gastrointestinal bleeding, and everyone over fifty should have an annual stool occult blood test.

The simple finding of microscopic blood in the urine leads to great success in bladder and kidney cancer, while $35 spent for an annual PSA blood test picks up most prostate cancer. A chest X-ray for smokers finds some lung cancers early.

Depression, life-threatening at any age, need not be so with current drugs and psychotherapy. Schizophrenia, no less life-threatening, can be calmed if patients faithfully take their drugs.

Pneumonia has lost its sting owing to the wide availability of flu shots and pneumonia shots. I seldom encounter it now, but if I do, a course of antibiotics clears it up promptly.

As I see my steady stream of senior patients, their main complaints are often about taxes and the high cost of travel insurance. Their main medical fear is the memory loss of dementia, which is quite common past the age of eighty-five. Yet even Alzheimer's yields in small ways to drugs.

These elderly patients often discuss death, sometimes with my urging. As I suggest that many of them will live past the age of ninety, they laugh when I say they had better develop some hobbies for their old age. They are, in an important way, winners at the game of life, with a proven track record of durability. No one will say they died young. It seems that if my senior patients don't get careless as they cross the busy main street in front of my office, we may keep our relationship going for some time yet.

One of my favourite patients had me howling when I said that researchers may find a way to stop the aging process. He replied, askance, "You mean no one is going to die? So where will I park my car?"

Logistical problems in treating the elderly

Dealing with elderly patients is known to be time-consuming. It can also be dangerous to life and limb and property. This aspect is very important in my practice because I treat many ambulatory patients over the age of eighty, and some over ninety. That is what happens when a twenty-seven-year-old family physician starts his practice seeing middle-age patients and thirty years go by. So, where do the delays happen?

> **THE WAITING ROOM:** Difficulties begin here because there is a fair chance that older patients will not hear their names called when their time has come, no matter how loudly my receptionist yells. They may, however, respond to someone else's name, creating a gridlock of wheelchairs and walkers at the entry, and an occasional shoving match with sharp words and sharper elbows.

> **LIFT OFF:** Some elderly people are extremely slow in rising from their chairs. In our office, my associate, whose patients are mainly young women, can get started on the consultation even before my patients have managed to stand up.

> **THE CARAVAN:** When the patient finally rises and begins hobbling toward my room, he or she may be accompanied by a spouse, a caretaker, and two daughters. A son brings up the rear, holding the oxygen tank. I smile sweetly and greet everyone politely while thinking, "This consultation should take a while." Patients in wide-body motorized wheelchairs may damage walls and doors en route. Once in the

examining room, parking these vehicles involves my moving furniture, and then each patient making several docking manoeuvres while I cringe against the wall.

POSITIONING OF THE PATIENT: One rather stubborn neurologically impaired patient has difficulty seating himself but rejects any assistance. He lowers himself into the chair so slowly that it appears he is not moving at all. Time stands still as his bottom won't budge until his wife comes to our rescue by administering the final push. Patients who cannot access the examining table can be examined in the chair, but this procedure is hard on the physician's back.

POSITIONING OF THE RETINUE: This group presents a logistical problem, and I do not like them hovering. If I don't have enough chairs, they sit on the examining table or on an unoccupied walker. It can be difficult staying focused if everyone has questions, and the patient may feel resentment if left out of the conversation, especially if deaf.

DISROBING: In winter, I find that the older patients dress in layers – lots of layers. I once counted six as I helped by lifting one garment up, then lowering the next, then raising the next, and so on. Even then I sometimes encounter an insurmountable obstacle on some of my female patients – an ancient girdle extending from bosom to the crotch, with clips below. Men present another kind of obstacle if they are wearing suspenders, which make it difficult to expose the chest.

THE PRELIMINARIES, INCLUDING THE DRUG DUMP: Elderly patients often come with a brown bag full of their medications. I never reach in, having learned from bitter experience what it may contain, so I dump the contents on my desk. Arthritic patients may not cap the bottles securely, so the pills wind up scattered on the floor. I then have to spend some time on my knees collecting them – truly a humbling experience. Many patients create an impossible dilemma by putting several different drugs in one labelled bottle – a problem that can be solved only if you can distinguish among several look-alike little white pills.

DEMENTIA OR DEPRESSION: If patients with these conditions have associated behaviour problems, watch out. One man had blackened the eyes of his caregiver and his wife, and I didn't want to be next. Another had left his antidepressant medication in Florida. After several days of withdrawal, he began chasing his wife, brandishing his cane. By the time he saw me, he was calmer, because I had reintroduced his drugs, but I was still wary. Canes are a special problem, and the only safe place for them is on the doorknob. Otherwise they fall and must be tiptoed around by both the patient and me. There are two other advantages to the doorknob placement: the cane will not be forgotten after the visit, and it will not be available as a weapon. Patients may react quite aggressively when we physicians have their driver's licences suspended or when we suggest it's time to move into a nursing home.

AFTER THE VISIT: With my head still swimming from all these problems, I hope after difficult consultations that my experienced secretary will present me with a younger patient, allowing me to regenerate myself. In family practice, however, we need to enjoy treating the elderly because they are the ones who keep us busy. I have, moreover, learned a lot from my elderly patients over the years, and we always leave a bit of time for the lighter stuff.

Driving while demented

This scenario is based on a story I read: A group of elderly patients were sitting in my waiting room, comparing ailments. "My arthritis is so bad I can't hold my coffee with my crippled hands, never mind turn my neck," said one lady. That comment inevitably invited a response from her neighbour: "Don't complain. My cataracts are so bad I can't even see my coffee." The second woman's flushed husband said, "I take so many blood-pressure pills I get dizzy and can barely stand up." A hearing-impaired gent leaned forward, inquiring, "What?" His pal answered: "Don't ask me what these ladies are talking about. Where am I, and how did I get here, and did we eat dinner yet?"

"Well, we should all count our blessings," said the first woman. "At least we can drive."

As physicians, we have a particular dilemma knowing when to pull the driving licence of all those patients. The urgent one to deal with is the last, the demented patient, leading to the dangerous habit of what I call DWD – driving while demented. It has been estimated that once dementia takes hold, drivers have a five-fold increase in accidents. Dementia can actually be given a number by using the MMSE – the mini mental-status exam – which is easily done during an office visit. We know that any score less than 30/30 might be a failure, if the test is done accurately, but do we act when the result is 25/30 or 20/30?

If possible when I encounter such patients, I seek an early consultation from a neurologist or a geriatric psychiatrist, who can make the decision to notify the Ministry of Transportation (MOT). That relieves me of incurring the eternal enmity of my patient. In one recent example, at their children's request, I sent one confused couple (Jon and Jane) down this route. Because their combined MMSE scores were 35/30, it was a no-brainer for the consultant to notify the MOT. He offered them redemption of their licences if they were able to pass a several-hour-long road test that cost hundreds of dollars. No one takes this expensive option, once appraised of likely failure.

Jane took to bed for forty-eight hours, sobbing that her independence was gone. Over that same period, Jon saw me twice and called me thrice, railing loudly against the injustice of it all. "I have never had an accident in fifty years of driving," he said. "How could you send us to that quack?" Then came the personal attack: "You tricked us into seeing him. You knew what he would do." Jon was almost right. I did know what might happen, but the referral was made to assess and treat their dementia. Driving abilities were secondary. I ignored the insult, knowing the tremendous anger Jon was demonstrating by lashing out. His children were other targets.

My advice to colleagues is to not refer both spouses at the same time for dementia or driving assessments. Refer the one who is in worse condition, let the results and the decisions sink in, and then proceed with the second referral as soon as it seems reasonable. If the second referral is refused by the spouse, the onus is then on the family physician to pull the licence and bear the brunt of the hostility that is almost sure to follow. A driving mishap causing personal injuries is much harder to bear, as is clear from the experience of another of my patients. In this case the driver, aged ninety-two, accelerated too fast as he pulled out of a shopping plaza, struck several empty parked cars, and came to a sudden stop when he smashed into another vehicle. When the airbags deployed, they fractured his frail wife's wrist. One passenger in the back seat sustained a fractured shoulder, and the other had neck injuries.

My patient surrendered his driver's licence to the investigating police officer. He does not seem to be demented, but perhaps his combination of arthritis, deafness, arrhythmia, and impaired reflexes led to the accident. I plan to assess him for dementia with some urgency because he has convinced his cardiologist that his licence should be renewed.

It certainly seems appropriate for authorities in Ontario to evaluate seniors' driving skills more thoroughly than they do at present through the written test administered to everyone over the age of eighty. On the law of averages, perhaps a third of the people eighty-five and older demonstrate some signs of dementia.

Vehicular attack – good golly, it's Dolly!

In my mind I saw my elderly patient Dolly limping along with her cane, moving slowly through deep snow. Blasted by winds and nearly frozen, she was dressed far too lightly for this blizzard. All she saw through the falling snow was chicken-wire fencing and the hulks of distant vehicles. Finally, at the end of the path was a shack. Encouraged, she put her head down and barrelled forward until she saw two men coming her way, rough-looking and unshaven. Would they help her or mug her? Both, as it turned out. Dolly had entered the Towing Zone, and she was at the mercy of greedy and opportunistic tow-truck drivers, a granny in big trouble – or so it seemed.

Like many elderly people, driving gave Dolly a measure of independence and self-esteem. No one gives it up without a fight. Her driving skills had been tested after she turned eighty, as is mandatory in Ontario. Still, I was doubtful after this incident that I had heard her entire story. Her account began at a doctor's office. She had an appointment and had arrived far too early, as elderly patients will. The only available parking was in a nearby restaurant lot, and she saw the notice "Cars will be towed after one hour." As often happens, she had to wait a while for the physician to see her, but she claimed she was finished before an hour had passed. When she returned to the parking lot, no car. Inquiries led to a phone call and the information she could retrieve her car for $154.

Dolly was frugal, so she took a bus rather than a taxi to the towing compound. She became confused in this unfamiliar territory and got off the bus too soon. Dressed for a drive, but not for a hike in a winter storm, she began her long walk. After thirty minutes, she stopped short when she saw the two men. They took her into the warm shack and explained their policy. The car would not be released until the money was paid. Dolly balked and insisted on calling the police, who said she had no choice but to pay. Still, she gave those men a strong argument and threatened to seek legal recourse – as well as place a curse on their progeny to the tenth generation. She later made them sorry they had ever been born, with her phone harassment, legal letters, and calls to supervisors and local politicians. Had they but realized what a dynamo they had snared, they would have paid her to take her car away. Dolly drove off quite rattled by the experience, muttering about her proposed retaliation, but she had calmed down when I saw her later that week.

She continued her disturbing narrative. A day after the towing, her vehicle was rear-ended and slightly damaged. Two days later she flooded the engine and again needed help. I am not at all a superstitious man, but I strongly believe that bad things happen in threes. Somewhat relieved, I told Dolly all was well: three incidents had already occurred, and she could carry on with impunity. She responded, "Not so fast, doctor dearest. Yesterday a stranger told me my car had a flat tire. So much for your theory of threes!" I didn't want to suggest that two more bad things must happen before Dolly could rest easy, but I did hint that she might be advised to stop driving. She almost yelled at me in response and waved her cane menacingly. Since then, she has stayed out of trouble, and she keeps passing her driving tests.

Family medicine, unlike some other specialties, is not limited to a single consultation – there may be many follow-up visits. The most recent one took place as I crossed a road near my office. I was startled to hear a loud honk, which propelled me to scoot out of a vehicle's way. It turned out to be Dolly's way of getting my attention. She pulled her car over and asked to be seen that afternoon. I couldn't say no to someone wielding so huge a weapon. I still cross the roads near my office very carefully. And I am quite sure there are two very uptight tow-truck operators also looking back over their shoulders lest an aged lady be stalking them with writ and cane and car.

Accident-prone people

Bad things can happen in elevators and on escalators, in airplanes and in ambulances. Who can expect in a hospital to be punched out in a corridor or sent flying by revolving doors? Apparently we are unsafe in casinos and bingo halls, and even in recreation centres if treadmills are available. When the injuries are not severe, patients and their physicians may find humour in these situations once the injuries have healed and the litigation is complete. The physician must not be the first one to smile at these stories – not until the unfortunate patient has safely left the office. Loud laughter coming from the doc and his staff as the patient is wrapping up to go is a no-no.

This story is about an older couple I will call the Btfsplks, Mr. and Mrs. Joe Btfsplk – with apologies to cartoonist Al Capp, whose *L'il Abner* strip was set in Dogpatch. In the funny pages, Joe was a jinx to himself and anyone nearby. In my office, he had a wife, with whom he seemed to live under a permanent rain cloud while the sun shone on everyone around them.

They are a diminutive couple, and Joe got bullied once in a hospital corridor. An agitated muscular in-patient, for no apparent reason, punched him out and knocked him flat as Mrs. B. screamed. The emergency room staff, who knew him well, found no damage of note.

The couple had both received treatment the previous month, after a large revolving door in the hospital entrance went berserk. Again, for no apparent reason, when they came to visit a hospitalized friend, it speeded up and whacked them both, propelling them ten feet out the door onto the road. Joe suffered a fractured shoulder.

In 2003 a major power failure affected much of the northeast section of the North American continent. Guess who got stuck in their condo's elevator for several hours? I narrowly missed the same fate when my office elevator died just as I was about to step into it after work. The Btfsplks spent an eternity pushing buttons in the dark and trying to phone out for help as the elevator got more stuffy and hot. When finally released they were dehydrated and exhausted and again taken to the hospital, this time without incident until Joe's wife fell out of the ambulance.

How can someone fall out of an ambulance? Mrs. B was tending to her benighted husband because, as usual, he was sicker than she was. The ambulance had stopped in front of the hospital, and the attendants had gingerly put him on a gurney and wheeled him into the hospital. They forgot about Mrs. B, who grew impatient. She was tiny, and she missed a step as she tried to disembark, fell on her outstretched hand, and broke her wrist. That is how you fall out of an ambulance.

I cannot say that it was Joe who landed a small plane upside down at Buttonville Airport during a solo training flight. That was another of my patients – a younger man who soon after left the country. He showed up in my office ten years later to say hello, proudly in a pilot's uniform.

Neither was it Joe and Mrs. B who were on an ascending escalator at Toronto's Eaton Centre when another of my patients fell backwards. He found it impossible to correct this position until a young man heard his wife screaming and saved him.

But it was Joe Btfsplk who suggested that his wife try the treadmill in the rec room of their building. She was poorly coordinated and awkward from all her previous injuries. She twisted the wrong dial and set the speed at the jogging level. Joe was somewhere else close by when she was flung high in the air by the treadmill and landed about five feet away, breaking not one but both shoulders. Joe rushed back to the room when he heard a loud thud, followed by his wife's cries.

In spite of their bad luck, Joe and his jinxed wife lived into their eighties and died of natural, non-traumatic causes. They were childless, and the family jinx ended with them.

ENDINGS – DOCTORS and PATIENTS

Firing a doctor, firing a patient, and transferring records

In my own office, a former patient who "fired" me months ago is now giving me the cold shoulder and averting her eyes when I look in her direction. This unpleasant situation has come about because, after many years as my patient, she switched her allegiance to my associate following some trivial dispute. This change is not surprising, really, considering that a family physician may see a patient scores of times over the years. We can't be on our best behaviour every time, and she objected to a remark I made in a weak moment about her "shopping list" of complaints.

Several other patients leave quietly every year. We usually learn about their decision when the new physicians send us a signed authorization for the transfer of their medical records. Patients can be very demanding and fickle, and the fact that so few leave my practice probably means that I am doing something right. My family physician colleagues often raise this issue when we get together at meetings. We ask plaintively, "Why do patients change physicians after many years, especially the ones for whom we have done the most?" We cannot understand why they leave, even when they benefit from our occasional diagnostic triumphs, such as the early diagnosis of cancer.

We don't miss those who have scored many points against our good nature over the years by insisting on same-day service, no matter how busy the office is at the time. They make frequent requests for unpaid telephone advice and prescription repeats, demand unnecessary house calls, and even abuse our secretarial staff. Some expect letters to employers or lawyers or insurance companies to be done gratis, with howls of protest over a modest invoice. Should such a person decide later to return to my office, I have supreme satisfaction when my secretary quotes our policy: "Sorry, we do not accept patients back into our practice once they have transferred to another physician." The respect is gone, for both the patient and the physician, once a patient leaves, and a reunion is ill-advised.

Luckily, we physicians can also "fire" patients if they become too difficult. We need to have the strength of character to do so before they do us even more harm. The process requires us to send a registered letter to these patients, with the offer to remain on duty for a period of three weeks – long enough to allow them all to find new (and sadly unfortunate) physicians.

How do we physicians handle the transfer of patient records? Most patients give the file undeserved mythic status. They see us scribbling or typing during every visit and observe us leafing through the sheets for lab work or other information. Yet I believe that any patient history can fit on a single page, outlining past health, family history, medications and drug allergies, and immunizations. Pertinent consultations and lab work add just a few more pages.

When the new physician receives such a summary from me, I can almost hear the sigh of relief. Seldom has anyone called asking for more information. I never charge the patient for this service because there are mixed emotions when patients transfer. It becomes very costly for patients if retiring physicians give all their records to a storage facility, which then makes the records available as photocopies or CDs. Most material that is copied is useless to the new physician, especially if it contains illegible office notes.

Records should never be given to the patient directly unless they are sealed, because medical terminology can be terrifying and confusing. The best example is the common expression SOB. It simply means that the patient has shortness of breath. It is not an indication of character; indeed, the wise physician never writes disparaging comments in the file. Snide remarks can return to haunt if they are analyzed later in a court of law.

How do family physicians replace losses among their patients? The usual source is referral from satisfied patients, which generally means that if your patients are old, the new arrivals will also be old. While younger persons refer their parents, the old never send their progeny. Still, there is always a special tingle at the first interview, as most physicians try to make a good impression, even if it becomes painfully obvious that Mr. New Patient is just as obnoxious as the unlamented Mr. Former Patient.

I will sometimes spare the previous physician the knowledge that a valued patient has deserted. Rather than ask for records, I start fresh. Important consultation notes can be had from the specialists still seeing the patient. All family physicians seem to know when patient A or B has not visited lately, so knowledge of the defection comes eventually in a gentler way.

I am not too shy to ask new patients why they switched doctors. The reasons given are often laughable. My younger sister, who has a nearby family practice of her own, once correctly diagnosed her elderly patient with a coronary thrombosis, drove him to the hospital in her car, and sat with him in the emergency department until the cardiologist arrived. This patient later left her practice because he preferred seeing a male doctor!

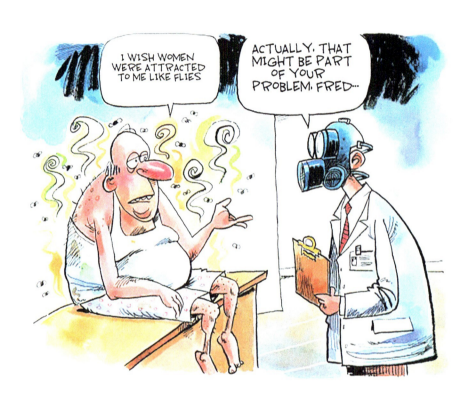

Olfactory adventures

I plead innocent in the firing of my patient Fred. It was complicated by the more acute sense of smell that women seem to have, compounded by the fact that I had lost much of my own such sense by then.

The situation arose in my packed waiting room. There sat chubby Fred with his arms crossed, elbowing the ladies on either side of him, both of whom seemed discomfited by this situation but unable to find another seat. Oddly, those patients who were standing were gathered in the farthest corner of the room. Fred smiled beatifically in the manner of those who never have too much on their minds.

In his forties on this last visit, Fred had never been a problem patient and would be the last to complain about a long wait. A doctor's visit was the highlight of his social life, and where else would he be in such close contact with women? Still, those two ladies beside him were clearly unhappy. Was he secretly tickling them with his hidden hands every time he moved? Not so, as things turned out.

As in any busy office, this trio had to wait quite a while, until my partner took me aside and said, "You must get rid of that guy – he has stunk up the whole office again. Call him in stat and keep the visit short!" I excused her brusqueness because a casual glance around the room showed that she and others looked as though they had just been sprayed by a skunk.

I called Fred in out of order, and no one complained. We did our medical business, and then I pointed out that he had ignored my previous attempts to teach him elementary hygiene. He understood why I had to fire him as a patient and left with my note of referral to his unspecified next physician.

Within a week I received a request for his records from a colleague downstairs, and a month later I saw the same waiting room tableau as I passed my friend's office. Fred's aroma was repelling other patients all the way to the outside hall. At our next medical rounds, my friend gave me a quizzical look, but I kept mum and played dumb when he thanked me for my notes on Fred.

This story brings me to a very embarrassing personal revelation – I get gas. This condition is not unusual because we all get gas that must be dealt with. In our profession the problem is exacerbated by the amount of talking and teaching we must do with our patients, one after the other, without a break, and with rare chances to use the washroom. It is possible to quietly relieve some of the pressure between patients while recording the visit, but that adds olfactory discomfort to the next patient. As a kindness to these people, I judiciously use an air freshener after every expulsion.

My chief proof of the possible damage comes from my wife. She is not shy about raising an unearthly howl about my efforts at home, accompanied by waiving her dishtowel around to clear the air. I know that women break wind too, but she is far more delicate about it. She has no tolerance for anything I produce, so it must be bad.

In our office, my "five o'clock flatus" has been known to produce an awkward situation for our medical secretaries at the end of the day. My first chance for a much-needed healthy release comes when the last patient has departed. I close my door, relax at my desk, and toot. Unfortunately, just after that comes a hesitant knock at my office door. My secretary can't go home until she gives me my messages, so she walks right into danger when I call her in. It could all be avoided if I sprayed my air freshener, but that would require expert coordination and timing from me. So it becomes a workplace hazard through which she carries on bravely, then flees.

As physicians age, so do our patients. Once their hearing and sense of smell go, they quite often launch clearly audible and disgusting explosions. They are unaware of this rude behaviour because they cannot hear or smell, so they must think I can't either. If they are demented, they don't care. Sometimes I spray the examining room and leave the door ajar for comfort and survival. The only solution is to toot back, and my secretaries may hear what sounds like World War III, a literal exchange of fire, coming from my examining room. Such episodes provide me with a justified opportunity to break wind during my busy day and cut down on the five o'clock flatus. Or so I hope.

NEW BEGINNINGS

Rating MDs – how to fight back

Misguided patients have begun asking me to refer them to physicians they had researched on the website RateMDs. I had never heard of the particular gastroenterologist or neurologist they requested, but nothing of that sort mattered to these patients. They liked the glowing comments that anonymous individuals had made, unaware that physicians can secretly post favourable ratings about themselves, as I once did.

Imagine if you will a doctor's lounge that is besieged by a mob of angry and critical patients who are hurling pill bottles and syringe-darts, epithets, insults, and curses at their cowering physician. Sadly, that is how some physicians feel after they have been hurt by awful criticisms found on RateMDs. Some have sued, but we can fight back in other ways – and have fun doing so.

When a physician googles himself now, he may be surprised to find RateMDs among the first entries he sees. With a few clicks, he may learn that some patients have a low opinion of him. Malicious people can ruin a doctor's reputation anonymously, and they may well outnumber the satisfied patients who have taken the time to write to the site.

In family practice, we see the same patients several times a year for decades, so we expect that, inevitably, we'll make a careless remark or decline the request for a prescription or a test at some time during our relationship with our regulars. After a conflict, if we check the website, we often find that patient's view of the visit described on the site. You cannot please everyone all the time.

One esteemed colleague's care over many years was summed up in these ungracious words: "She made an incorrect diagnosis, she was rude and rushed, and as I left she made fun of me. To add insult to injury, she told her secretary to bill me $20 for a note it took her twenty seconds to write."

My own negative ratings are pretty tame:

- "All he does is shake his head and says 'See me in three months.'"
- "He is disinterested in the patient and mainly interested in talking about his vacations."
- "Makes you wait 1.5 hours even when you have a scheduled appointment. I left twice without seeing him. Will not return."

Some physicians have responded by submitting favourable comments and ratings about themselves. As an experiment while on holiday I did just that, four times in a short period of time, each one 999 characters long, the maximum allowed. One of them read, "I wood [sic] give Dr. Rapoport full marks but an explination is needed. He nagged me to death over a long period of time about my cigrettes and licker, but he finally got threw to me …"

All four submissions were deleted within three weeks, not for bad grammar and spelling but because they were "positive duplicate or disallowed ratings automatically removed." I had sent them all from the same computer. Any creative colleague can get around this problem by sending paeans of praise from computers in the homes of friends and relatives.

I saw some frightening write-ups in RateMDs about me from people who objected to a letter I had sent to the editor of a newspaper. These missives did not belong on the site because they were not written by patients, and I got them removed by appealing to the site managers.

As a service to readers who are my patients and who wish to rate me in the various categories on the site, I have composed a list of synonyms I found in my thesaurus. They also apply to colleagues who want to have some fun:

- Knowledge: Please avoid *ignorant* and *clueless*. Choose from *well informed, on the ball, conversant, familiar, expert*, and *experienced*.
- Helpfulness: Please avoid *useless, apathetic, inattentive, daydreaming*, and *distracted, blasé, aloof*, and *remote, negligent*, and *remiss*. I prefer *obliging, supportive and caring, effective and cooperative*.
- Punctuality: Avoid *tardy, late*, and the frequently paraphrased *He couldn't care less that I waited ninety minutes*. Select from *on time, prompt, on the dot*, or you might say, *He is worth waiting for*.

If we send duplicates and flood the site in this manner, we will certainly improve our score to five out of five in each category. We may also attract enough attention from the executives of RateMDs, who may do the right thing and declare that writers must identify themselves when writing about their physicians. With anonymity lost, our problem is solved. End of story.

Electronic medical records

Imagine if you will a senior physician struggling to use his new electronic medical records (EMRs) system just after it "goes live." He may not know it yet, but he is now completely under the control of a malevolent computer program called Oscar. His life will never be the same again, as he will learn with the first patient he sees. He has willingly entered this Twilight Zone where he will find no mercy and where there is no easy way out except retirement.

As his long-term patient, what can you do if you're alone with your physician when the kindly old doc finally flips out? These are common scenarios, so beware.

You enter his waiting room and see an unruly mob scene, with lots of unhappy grumblers looking at their watches. You sit for ninety minutes without spotting his secretary. Deep in the office you hear your soft-spoken doc and Maria, his quietly devoted secretary, yelling loudly at each other about computers and printers.

When Maria finally pokes her nose out to call you in, she is a mess – tearful, frazzled, and exasperated, hair wild as she shakes her head in disbelief. She whispers, "He is in a bad mood today because Oscar won't cooperate. Keep the visit short if you can. Call me in if you need help."

You finally enter his examining room, and he is visibly unhappy. There is no eye contact once he starts pecking away at his keyboard. Ten minutes pass as he painstakingly prescribes each of your ten drugs – doses, amounts, and repeats for each one – then proudly demonstrates his finesse to you by pushing a button. In an instant, all of his work disappears. His frustration is enormous. He grabs a pen and writes the prescriptions longhand, as in the old days – last week – all in just two minutes.

He turns to the printer to print something. The printer spits out twenty-five blank pages as the doc tries frantically to halt the beast – unplugging the machine at the wall or turning it off seems the only solution. He phones the hardware supplier and is told to remove the paper from the printer to stop this madness, give it five minutes' rest, then try again.

He explains to you that with EMRs he can do nothing without a functioning printer, which is needed several times each visit to do lab requisitions, prescriptions, and referrals. After a distracted chat with you for those five minutes he tries to print again, only to see the monster resume spewing out blanks until it jams up. He is in a pitiable state by then, moaning "I give up."

He hunts fruitlessly for the lab work and imaging you had done just a week ago. These tests are the reason for today's follow-up visit, after all, so he yells at his secretary to find them in the electronic ether. Maria has had enough abuse by then, so she yells back and phones the lab and X-ray staff to yell at them. The results are actually in the office, but they have not yet been scanned into the documents section of the patient's e-file. The doctor mutters that it's no different from the old days – last week – when staff got behind with the paper filing.

So you, the patient, become the therapist, trying unsuccessfully to calm the doctor down as he paces around the small examining room, smacking the computer and the printer on each circuit. When he picks up the keyboard and tries to smash it in half across his knee, you run out to Maria for help. She tells you she has already called 911. You are happy to leave.

Disclosure: This story is of course exaggerated. I'm pleased to report that in my office, eighteen months after "going live," things were humming along nicely for me. I never became quite as disturbed as the doc in my tale – physicians learn to hide a lot of stress in front of their patients. My always calm and efficient secretary Maria kept a lid on things during my tantrums, as always, and without a bad-hair day.

When the dust settled, Oscar pointed out that many of these problems were user errors, and they disappeared after I got further training by his minions. Oscar's software people agreed to install a more powerful wireless system, and the weekly meltdowns soon disappeared. The printer's bad habit of regurgitating multiple sheets has been resolved. Oscar has won: I am effectively in his power and happy about it.

Capitation and its temptations

Many family physicians in Ontario are members of Family Health Organizations (FHOs), which are based on a roster of patients. Our fees are set according to a capitation system, and we are paid monthly by the Ministry of Health and Long-Term Care (MOHLTC). With the demise of fee-for-service, physicians find that the volume of patients we actually see in the office can be much reduced.

If patients are not seen, we don't order lab work and imaging, we don't prescribe, and we don't make referrals. Many authorities feel that these costly interventions are done too often in any case. Patients are already monitoring their own blood pressure and glucose at home and can be asked to call if the results are abnormal. They have many other options in our healthcare system, including our mandated after-hours clinic staffed by real humans.

With the help of electronic medical records (EMRs) and Oscar, my robotic e-nurse practitioner, I am able to keep office visits to a minimum. Knowing my password, he has access to every caller's e-file and cumulative patient profile (CPP). He has an encyclopedic knowledge of all things medical, including drugs, and he bases his functional inquiry on available modules in the SOAP (subjective, objective, assessment, and plan) format. He records all contacts in the e-files.

I will admit that, being updated daily, he knows more than I do about everything. Still, he is under my supervision, and I follow each contact remotely, in real time or later in the day. His somewhat sarcastic phone etiquette can be a bit problematic, but we are working on that. He can raise his voice when necessary to a degree I control.

Oscar has been trained to discourage unnecessary office visits by using my voice mail, email, and Skype. For patients who he thinks need to be seen in the office, he books an appointment at a time when I am available for backup and physical examinations. He knows in nanoseconds if the caller is overdue for preventive measures and arranges mammography, Pap smears, and bone density tests according to the current guidelines, every two or three years.

Over the phone he offers patients advice about colds, asthma, influenza, and bladder infections. If it is a simple matter of renewing antibiotics or inhalers that helped previously, Oscar can do so after perusing the e-file. If he learns that the patient is a smoker with chronic obstructive pulmonary disease (COPD), Oscar can raise his voice and get pretty nasty – I trained him that way.

For sexual problems, for males with STDs, he delivers a stern lecture as well as a hefty course of antibiotics, after examining the genitals via Skype. I have allowed him to yell in this situation as well, especially if the cringing caller is married. In that case Oscar swears himself to secrecy. The patient is told that his partner will never hear of this consultation. For females he renews medications such as birth control pills and antifungals after taking a brief history. If a pelvic exam is needed, he will arrange it by me or by the caller's gynecologist.

Oscar can handle some emotional problems. He starts by asking if the caller is suicidal, and if so he advises going immediately to the nearest ER. He can send an ambulance if needed. For those seriously depressed but not suicidal, Oscar can perform twice-weekly psychotherapy or cognitive behavioural therapy and, if needed, prescribe the appropriate medications. He follows the available depression module until I or a psychiatrist takes over. For the mildly neurotic, he will take a detailed history, then suggest that the patient get a life and stop bothering us.

Requests to see specialists other than family physicians are referred to me only if Oscar deems them necessary after a discussion with the patient. That eliminates the 90 percent of such requests he handles himself. He acts as a gatekeeper but will send a required referral request if he's convinced the patient needs one. In some cases the specialist is already seeing the patient regularly for diabetes, heart disease, arthritis, and other chronic conditions.

Oscar can handle most skin problems and rashes via Skype through his dermatologist app. After checking the entire body, he will ask the patient to expose the area involved. He is not offended by armpits or crotches, even if the patient needs to "moon" him. If he sees something really suspicious or ugly, he will refer the patient to a dermatologist.

I see every patient at least once a year, after Oscar has taken a complete functional inquiry and scanned in the current lab work and consultations. I review all this material and do a brief physical examination. I have been able to lease a smaller office and let all my human staff go. Oscar works for free, never gets pregnant or sick, and works 24/7. Patients are happy with the instant attention, and the MOHLTC is thrilled to save hundreds of thousands of dollars every year.

About the author

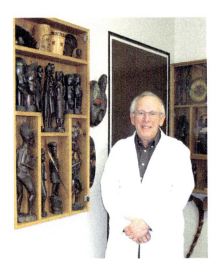

Dr. David Rapoport was born in Toronto and graduated in medicine from the University of Toronto. He has practised family medicine in North Toronto since 1969 and believes that over all that time the unique doctor-patient relationship has remained much the same.

For more than twenty years, he has been writing about the lighter side of medicine in the former *Family Practice* and in *Medical Post*, both medical newsmagazines. *Medical Post* eventually took over *Family Practice*, and it is now part of the Canadian Healthcare Network. Each of these magazines devoted its last page to medical humour, with an illustration by a talented artist. Dr. Rapoport also wrote in *Stitches*, another medical humour magazine. In one banner week around 2000 he had articles in all three publications. He insists he is not responsible for the demise of *Family Practice* and *Stitches*.

Dr. Rapoport says that most of his patients can be assessed in a light-hearted way because they appreciate a little humour. In turn, they have taught him a lot on the subject. Favourite patients bring laughter into many a long day, and patients in the waiting room hear it. They either wonder what's going on or are annoyed that they must wait even longer. Physicians know they may have to switch attitudes for the next patient, who could have a grim diagnosis.

In addition to writing, Dr. Rapoport's hobbies include woodworking, a skill practised by a grandfather from England; collecting African wood-carvings, mainly bought at garage sales; playing golf with similarly inept duffers; crosswords, and what he calls his "Ritual Sudoku."

Acknowledgements

I am very grateful to my son Mark, who, by teaching me computer word processing, set my imagination free, and to my son Jonathan, whose expertise keeps my office and home machines humming along. My wife, Sharon, is well versed in computer programs and has rescued me many times from the depths of despair when I am stymied by a computer glitch. She is also my private photographer.

The editors of the various medical publications in which my stories have appeared have been very kind with their helpful suggestions. They include Simon Hally of *Stitches*, Vil Meere and Elaine McNinch of *Family Practice*, and Joe McAllister, David Hodges, Leo Charbonneau, Jacob Rutka, Carole Hilton, Rick Campbell, and Colin Leslie of *Medical Post*. Acceptance of a story by phone or by email always makes my day and gives me several weeks of happy anticipation until the letter carrier arrives with the actual publication.

I also thank the artists who so capably illustrated some of the stories, especially Peter Cook, Tom Goldsmith, Dave Prothero and Dave Whamond, who have graciously allowed me to publish their work. A special thanks goes to *National Post* cartoonist Gary Clement, for his art work on my late mother Rose as a waiting room spy, the illustration used as the front cover art for this book.

In preparing these stories for publication in this book, I have revised some of the texts, changed some of the original titles, and grouped the stories by theme. I have made numerous changes, including to gender, to ensure patient confidentiality, and the March of Time has done the rest. I have been practising medicine for over forty-five years, so many of the older patients I write about are, unfortunately, deceased.

When I was encouraged to gather these stories into one publication, I was recommended to Rosemary Shipton, who agreed to be my editor. She in turn introduced me to designers Peter Ross and Linda Gustafson of Counterpunch Inc. I want to thank them all, as well as proofreader Judy Phillips, for their work in producing this book.

Credits

Some of the stories have been published previously (often under different titles) in the *Canadian Medical Association Journal*, *Family Practice*, the *Medical Post*, and *Stitches*, and publication dates are included here if they are available. For illustrations, the artist's name is included where it is known; for illustrations included in this book, the artist's name is in boldface. The stories that have not been published include the year in which I wrote them.

Staff

Staff – our first line of defence (2013, illustrated by **Tom Goldsmith**)
Hurricane Mabel – my mixed-up medical secretary (*Family Practice* 1995, illustrated by Andy)
Medical secretary required – ideal qualifications (*Medical Post* 1999, illustrated by Tom Goldsmith; 2013)

Waiting-room adventures

Waiting, waiting, and more waiting – ten patients behind (*Family Practice* 1997, illustrated by **Andy**)
A demented duo takes over the waiting room (*Family Practice* 1997, illustrated by Andy)
Patients who fight (*Family Practice* 1997)
Thumps in the waiting room (*Medical Post* 2004, illustrated by Joe Weissman)
Drop-in Bob (*Medical Post* 2012, illustrated by Dave Whamond)

In the examining room

Goofy about gonads (*Medical Post* 2000, illustrated by **Tom Goldsmith**)
The rear admiral (*Family Practice* 1996)
The window washer and the pelvic exam (*Medical Post* 2005)
Belly laughs (*Family Practice* 1997)
Punmeister (*Medical Post* 1997, illustrated by Tom Goldsmith)
Emergencies – firefighters, police officers, and ambulance attendants (2013)
Lying in state in the doctor's office (2014)
The gamblers (Bingo, *Medical Post* 1999; other stories 2002 and 2012)

Abominations and embarrassing situations

How to make your physician remember you (*Family Practice* 1995)
How to make your patients remember you (2003)

Tools of the trade

Doctors causing high blood pressure (*Stitches* 1998)
The stethoscope – the colder the better (2013)
The many uses of the humble tongue depressor (*Medical Post* 1995)
The nerd pocket (2013)

Peculiar patients

Doorknobs, handshakes, and other hazards (*Family Practice* 1996, illustrated by **Dave Prothero**)
Examining-room ballet (*Medical Post* 2012, illustrated by Dave Whamond)
Fainters, grabbers, and smoochers (*Stitches* 1995, with a follow-up in *Medical Post* 2013)
The carrot people (*Family Practice* 1997, illustrated by Dave Prothero)
Whistlers and hummers (1996)

Physicians' bad habits

Performing ritual Sudoku in medical practice (*Medical Post* 2006, photo by Sharon Rapoport)
The five-pound Hershey bar (*Medical Post* 2000, photo by Sharon Rapoport)
Snoozing sickness (*Stitches* 1995; *Medical Post* 2005)
Snoozing physicians (*Globe and Mail* blog 2013)
Doctors who yell (*Family Practice* 1998)
Hiccups (*Medical Post* 1998)

Mind games
Beware of honest physicians – they may be dangerous (1997)
Bizarre coincidences in medical practice (2000)
Deconstructing Michelangelo's *David* (2004)

Drug reps, drug companies, and prescription pads
Drug reps bearing flattery, adulation, and praise (*Medical Post* 1997, illustrated by **Tom Goldsmith**)
Drug companies bearing gifts (*Canadian Medical Association Journal* 1995)
Drug dreams (*Family Practice* 1999, illustrated by **Dave Prothero**)
A daring method of drug selection for the harried family physician (*Medical Post* 2004)
Goldilocks revisited (1997)
Reconstructing Mary (2003)
My polydoctor patient (*Family Practice*)
A cautionary tale about vultures, fish, snakes, and devils on drugs (2013)

Meeting patients outside the office
House calls – how to handle dogs, doors, and defunct doorbells (*Medical Post* 2009)
Lessons in patient avoidance (*Medical Post*)
The beach, the mall, and the wedding hall (*Medical Post* 1996, illustrated by **Craig Terison**)
Is there a doctor on the plane? (*Medical Post* 2013)

Doctors get sick too
Coronary heart disease (*Medical Post* 1991, 2000, 2010–13, photo by Sharon Rapoport)
Sleep apnea (*Medical Post* 2008, photo by Sharon Rapoport)

Baseball as metaphor for the practice of medicine
Doctors and baseball pitchers must get the opponent out (*Medical Post* 2003, illustrated by **Peter Cook**)

A new seasonal affective disorder (*Medical Post* 2011, 2012, illustrated by **Dave Whamond**)

Body image and plastic surgery
The widow's facelift (*Stitches* 1996)
Why plastic surgery patients switch doctors (1995)
My nude dye job (*Medical Post* 2003)
Bald and balder – or a tale of two drug reps (*Medical Post* 1998, illustrated by Craig Terlson)
Big-belly syndrome (*Medical Post* 2014, illustrated by **Dave Whamond**)

Sex
Fleeing from temptation (1998)
Viagra – making sex fun at any age (*Medical Post* 2008)

Parents and elderly patients
My parents – our waiting-room spies (*Medical Post* 1996, illustrated by **Gary Clement**; *Medical Post* 2007, photo by Sharon Rapoport)
Death takes a holiday (2004)
Logistical problems in treating the elderly (*Family Practice* 1998, illustrated by Andy)
Driving while demented (2004)
Vehicular attack – good golly, it's Dolly! (*Medical Post* 1996)
Accident-prone people (*Medical Post* 2001)

Endings – doctors and patients
Firing a doctor, firing a patient, and transferring records (2013 and *Family Practice*, 1997)
Olfactory adventures (*Medical Post* 2013, illustrated by **Dave Whamond**)

New beginnings
Rating MDs – how to fight back (*Medical Post* 2011)
Electronic medical records (2013)
Capitation and its temptations (2013)

CPSIA information can be obtained at www.ICGtesting.com
Printed in the USA
LVOW05s0410150715

446098LV00029B/256/P

9 780994 089502